DOCTORS AND THE STATE

The Making of Modern Africa

Series Editors: Abebe Zegeye and John Higginson

Doctors and the State

The struggle for professional control in Zimbabwe

DOROTHY MUTIZWA-MANGIZA

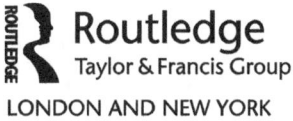

Routledge
Taylor & Francis Group

LONDON AND NEW YORK

First published 1999 by Ashgate Publishing

Reissued 2018 by Routledge
2 Park Square, Milton Park, Abingdon, Oxon OX14 4RN
711 Third Avenue, New York, NY 10017, USA

Routledge is an imprint of the Taylor & Francis Group, an informa business

Publisher's Note
The publisher has gone to great lengths to ensure the quality of this reprint but points out that some imperfections in the original copies may be apparent.

Disclaimer
The publisher has made every effort to trace copyright holders and welcomes correspondence from those they have been unable to contact.

A Library of Congress record exists under LC control number: 99072335

ISBN 13: 978-1-138-61839-8 (hbk)
ISBN 13: 978-1-138-61841-1 (pbk)
ISBN 13: 978-0-429-46122-4 (ebk)

Contents

List of Figures and Tables

Acknowledgements

I wish to express my gratitude to the World Bank Scholarship Programme for awarding me a two-year scholarship to complete the research on which this book is based and the Department of Sociology, University of Zimbabwe, for granting me leave of absence. My most particular gratitude goes to Dr. Ellen Annandale, my PhD supervisor in the Department of Sociology, University of Warwick, for her guidance and unwavering support. I want to gratefully thank the many doctors and key informants whom I cannot name individually, but who gave so generously of their time and information. Many thanks to my dear friends who supported and encouraged me: my mentor, Professor Robin Cohen and his wife Selina; Lou Ann Barclay; Angela Bacchus and Clara Mufuka, with whom I shared a dream but who did not live long enough to realise their own; Mwaiti Sibanda; Rudo Gaidzanwa; Martha Nyazema; Rose Munangatire; Tendai Mutangadura; Florence and Ben Sambana; Joyce Kazembe; Mary Maboreke; Sipho Moyo; Mildred Mkandla; and Agnes Runganga.

   I would like to thank the clan for their love and encouragement: my sisters Rufaro, Rutendo, Margaret, Chiri Doreen, and brothers Lenson and Taruvedza; Norah Zenda, my grandmother, Herida Zenda my great-aunt and Winnie Zenda my loving aunt; the first and greatest teachers in my life, my parents Idah and Enoch Mirimi Zenda (Chief Svosve wa Gahadza) who taught me that anything is possible with hard work and discipline and whose strong belief in education spurred me to work hard.

   A special tribute to my children, Shingai and Chiedza, for their unconditional love, resilience and for suppressing evidence of 'maternal deprivation'. Most of all, I wish to thank my soul mate and best friend, Naison, who made it possible for me to pursue and realise my dream. I thank him for his unwavering love, moral and financial support, for reading drafts of this book and for being 'mom-dad' to our two children while I was away. Last, but not least, my sincere gratitude to Anne Idukitta for preparing the camera-ready copy of this book. I dedicate this book to my husband, Naison, and our two children, Shingai and Chiedza.

Dorothy Mutizwa-Mangiza
Nairobi, Kenya

List of Abbreviations

AMA — American Medical Association
BMA — British Medical Association
CIMAS — Commercial and Industrial Medical Aid Society
CPCP — College of Primary Care Physicians
CSSD — Central Sterilising Supplies Department
DRG — Diagnostic Related Groups
ECG — Electro-cardiograph
EDLIZ — Essential Drugs List of Zimbabwe
ESAP — Economic Structural Adjustment Programme
GMC — General Medical Council
HDA — Hospital Doctors Association
HMO — Hospital Medical Officer
HPC — Health Professions Council
IMF — International Monetary Fund
JHDA — Junior Hospital Doctors Association
JRMO — Junior Resident Medical Officer
MOH — Ministry of Health (renamed MOH & CW in 1990)
MOH & CW — Ministry of Health and Child Welfare
MRB — Medical Responsibility Board
NAMAS — National Association of Medical Aid Societies
NHS — National Health Service
RMA — Rhodesia Medical Association
RMC — Rhodesia Medical Council
SDF — Social Development Fund
SHO — Senior House Officer
SRC — Scientific Research Council
SRMO — Senior Resident Medical Officer
UDI — Unilateral Declaration of Independence
UNICEF — United Nations Children's Fund
ZACH — Zimbabwe Association of Church Related Hospitals
ZANU (PF) — Zimbabwe African National Union (Patriotic Front)
ZAPU (PF) — Zimbabwe African People's Union (Patriotic Front)
ZCTU — Zimbabwe Congress of Trade Unions

ZEDUP	Zimbabwe Essential Drugs Action Programme
ZIMCORD	Zimbabwe Conference on Reconstruction and Development
ZINA	Zimbabwe Nurses Association
ZINATHA	Zimbabwe National Traditional Healers Association
ZMA	Zimbabwe Medical Association

1 Introduction

The Problem and its Background

In November 1988, Zimbabwean society was shocked when junior doctors employed at its four central hospitals went on strike, the first ever by doctors in the history of the country. The strike lasted three days, after which, following negotiations with the government, the doctors went back to work. On the surface, it appeared that the causes of the strike had been adequately addressed in the negotiations. But to the public's surprise, six months later, in June 1989, the junior doctors once again came out on strike. This strike, which was closely reported in the media, pointed to underlying problems between the medical profession and government.

Even though it was only junior doctors who came out on strike, their senior colleagues working at government hospitals lent their support. Private medical practitioners sent a delegation to the country's President asking him to secure the release of junior doctors arrested during the strike. This united front was quite unusual, considering the deep divisions and conflicts that have historically been evident between the different sections of the medical profession in Zimbabwe.

When after the strike, doctors were given call duty, housing and transport allowances for the first time ever, it appeared as if the concerns which precipitated the strike had finally been settled. However, media reports indicated that there was still widespread dissatisfaction, manifest in the high turnover rates of junior and middle level doctors from government hospitals, which had reached an unprecedented 39 per cent in 1991 (*Herald*, February 17, 1992). Most junior and middle level doctors left government hospitals for neighbouring countries, such as Botswana and the South African homelands, which offered more attractive working conditions, while others went to join the ranks of the solo-fee-for service private practitioners within the country. The resultant shortage of doctors prevented the government from realising its planned staffing levels, particularly in the rural areas where it has been forced to rely even more heavily on expatriate doctors who neither understand the language nor the culture of the indigenous Zimbabweans.

Throughout the 1990s, the medical profession in Zimbabwe has hardly been out of the media and public focus. Besides the issue of attrition from public institutions, the medical profession has been kept in the spotlight by a malpractice suit brought against a senior private anaesthetist, Dr McGowan. The public outcry at the allegations levelled against him resulted in the appointment of a Parliamentary Select Committee in 1992 to investigate the regulation of the medical profession by the Health Professions Council (HPC), the body responsible for regulating all registrable health workers. The findings of the Parliamentary Select Committee led policy-makers, local and international human rights organisations, and members of the public to call for closer scrutiny and regulation of medical practice in the country (*Parliamentary Debates*, 20 October, 1993; 2 and 3 November, 1993).

Public focus on the medical profession has been further intensified by allegations that government-employed doctors spend too much time on their private patients during working hours at the expense of government patients. Clearly, the persistent problems which the Zimbabwe government has experienced since the 1988 strike signal the need for an in-depth critical analysis of the medical profession. Virtually nothing has been written on the medical profession in Zimbabwe, particularly with respect to its relationship to the state. This book, which analyses the nature of professional autonomy exercised by government-employed doctors in post-colonial Zimbabwe, aims to bridge this gap in sociological knowledge.

The aim of this chapter is to provide an analytical framework for the book. It begins by describing the nature of the problems which the Zimbabwe government has experienced with its medical employees, focusing on post-independence government health policies and the reaction of the medical profession and also drawing comparisons with other countries which adopted similar policies. The chapter then outlines the aims and rationale of the thesis, before discussing the conceptual framework which guided the study. Theorists of professions emphasize the centrality of the role of the state in determining the nature and degree of autonomy exercised by the medical profession in any society. Accordingly, the chapter proceeds to analyze the Zimbabwean state, highlighting its administrative, economic and social structures and the role of international finance agencies on government policies.

The Medical Profession and the State

A review of literature on the medical profession in countries such as Chile (Chanfreau, 1979); Nicaragua (Garfield and Williams, 1989); Britain (Forsyth, 1976; Garpenby, 1989; Klein, 1989) provided the idea that the underlying causes of the problems between the medical profession and the Zimbabwe government lay with the impact of some post-colonial health care policies on medical interests. Experiences of other countries indicate that the medical profession almost consistently opposes any policies that it perceives as potentially inimical to its interests. As Mechanic (cited in Alford, 1975: 9) points out, 'groups are usually reluctant to yield rights and privileges that they have already exercised and will resist significant restructuring unless it appears that there is something in it for them'.

The government which came to power in Zimbabwe at independence in 1980 was socialist-oriented and took a more radical and directive approach to health care than its colonial predecessor. Where the colonial government had presided over a health care system fragmented along racial, economic, geographical and provider lines, the post-colonial government expressed its commitment to the establishment of a unified, racially desegregated and egalitarian health care system, and proposed policies to achieve these objectives. These included: free health care for those earning the government-stipulated minimum wage of Z$150 per month or less; legalization of traditional medicine; review of medical education; curtailing private medicine; the introduction of an essential drugs list; and a bonding contract for locally educated physicians.

The leadership of the medical profession, that is the Rhodesia Medical Association (RMA), which was aware of the potential impact of such policies from the experiences of colleagues in Zambia, was apprehensive of the impact which the radical policies of a black government would have on medical practice even before independence in 1980 (cf. Cohen Committee, 1978). Specifically, the nationalisation of private health institutions which took place in Zambia after independence reduced the scope of private practice to private company facilities only (Cohen Committee, 1978), while Cuba lost more than 50 per cent of its medical profession to the United States when Castro's government came to power in 1959 (Garfield and Williams, 1989). In Chile, the medical profession was heavily implicated in the *coup d'etat* in which Allende was killed in 1972 (Chanfreau, 1979).

A policy of free health care for those earning the government stipulated minimum wage of Z$150 or less was introduced in Zimbabwe in September 1980 (MOH, 1984). This policy had the potential of reducing the market for private medical practice as most poor patients would utilise government health institutions where they did not have to pay for health care.

In 1981, the Witchcraft Act of 1899 which had curtailed the activities of traditional healers, such as divining, was repealed and the healers were recognised by government for the first time through the Traditional Medical Practitioners' Act (1981). This recognition and legitimisation also had the potential of reducing the market for private medical practice as the traditional healers could now employ all their diagnostic and treatment methods openly without fear of prosecution. However, the arduous experiences of paramedical workers and alternative healers in negotiating boundaries of competence and responsibility with the medical profession in Britain (Larkin, 1983, 1995) highlights potential problems for traditional healers seeking to secure their own niche in the Zimbabwean health market.

The new government attacked the country's medical education system, which was seen as elitist and unsuitable for equipping graduates with the skills necessary for dealing with the diseases prevalent in a developing country. The first post-colonial Minister of Health, Dr Ushewokunze, called for an increase in the medical school intake to meet the country's medical staffing needs (Ushewokunze, 1984). Gish and Martin (1979) argue that the medical profession in developing countries vehemently opposes suggestions of curriculum change which are intended to reflect the medical conditions of their own countries, preferring instead a curriculum which equips them for registration and employment in developed countries. Similarly, the medical profession is opposed to calls for increases in medical school intakes, as the profession is better able to negotiate for higher economic rewards when there is a national shortage of physicians (Gish, 1971).

The first post-independence Minister of Health also announced the government's opposition to private medicine and private health institutions. He explained that existing private health institutions would be allowed to continue operating, but the government would not allow further expansion of the sector since it allegedly prejudices the public sector (Ushewokunze, 1984; MOH, 1984). Experiences in other countries such as Chile (Chanfreau, 1979), Nicaragua (Garfield and Williams, 1989) and Britain

(Yates, 1995) have shown that the issue of private medicine is highly contested. The existence of a viable private medical sector gives the profession a choice to practise privately, whether on a full or part-time basis, and to earn extra income and as can be expected, any attempts by a government to tamper with this are vigorously resisted. For example, the British Medical Association (BMA) spent a considerable amount of money lobbying against the introduction of the National Health Service in the 1940s on the basis of expectations that it would seriously reduce opportunities for private practice (Forsyth, 1973; Klein, 1989). Similarly, the opposition of the American Medical Association has also been blamed for the lack of a national health insurance system in the United States (Alford, 1975; Starr, 1982; Freidson, 1988).

Most welfare or socialist-oriented governments are concerned to ensure that health care is accessible to all citizens regardless of their socio-economic status and to achieve this, they strive to ensure that the health infrastructure, resources and personnel are equitably distributed in the country, something which may interfere with physicians' ability to earn extra income. In its desire to redress the imbalance in the distribution of medical personnel between urban and rural areas and between the public and the private sector, the Zimbabwe government introduced a new employment contract (bonding) for medical graduates in 1987. Henceforth, locally trained medical graduates had to work in government for five years after a two year internship before they could leave government service.

In 1985, the Ministry of Health introduced an essential drugs list in a bid to control the cost of drugs, to reduce the waste of scarce foreign currency through unregulated importation of drugs, and to rationalise therapeutic procedures in government hospitals. Freidson (1988) states that the medical profession prefers a situation where clinical decisions are based solely on the clinical condition of the patient rather than on non-medical considerations. Consequently, the profession is opposed to any policies that attempt to limit its choices in the clinical decision-making process. For example, the medical profession in Great Britain was opposed to the introduction of a limited drugs list in 1985, even though this had little impact on their prescription practices (Elston, 1991; Harrison and Schulz, 1989; Klein, 1989).

Why is the relationship of the state and the medical profession central to this book? The experiences of other countries which have been pointed to in the above discussion partly provide an answer to that question. Their experiences suggest that the problems which the Zimbabwe

5

government is experiencing originate from the impact of some of its policies on the autonomy of the medical profession, and points to the need to examine its relationship with the profession closely. An examination of that relationship is germane, given that most of the problems are occurring in government institutions in which the state relies on doctors in the organisation and delivery of health care to the general population. In addition, all theorists of professions agree that the autonomy which the medical profession so jealously guards and which is the subject of this enquiry is granted by the state which continues to secure it (Dent, 1995; Freidson, [1970a], 1988; Hugman, 1991; Johnson, 1972, 1995; Larkin, 1983, 1995; Starr, 1982). Freidson (1970b:83) states, 'the foundation on which analysis of a profession must be based is its relationship to the ultimate source of power and authority in modern society - the state'. In a similar vein, Johnson (1972) noted that the state acts as a mediator between the professions and the clientele by defining who the clientele should be and the manner and the extent to which they should be helped. Accordingly, professions can only define their clientele within parameters agreed with the state, and similarly, professional responsibilities and prerogatives are restricted to areas delineated by the state through various legal frameworks, including licensing. The state also plays a mediative role between the various professional interests and has considerable control and influence over the structure, form and content of caring professions (Hugman, 1991; Johnson, 1972).

Aims and Objectives of the Book

The aim of this book is to explore the nature and extent of medical autonomy among government employed physicians in post-colonial Zimbabwe. The book adopts the conceptualisation of dimensions of medical autonomy and dominance identified by Freidson ([1970a], 1988) and Elston (1977, 1991), that is: the profession's control over the technical aspects of its work (clinical autonomy); terms and conditions of work (economic autonomy); collective regulation of medical education, licensing and medical discipline (collective autonomy or self regulation); and dominance. Freidson (1988) defines autonomy as the right to self-determination which an occupation exercises over some aspects of its work. As he points out, the most strategic distinction between professions and other occupations lies in legitimate and organised autonomy which the former enjoy. Medical

6

dominance and medical autonomy have often been used interchangeably, but for purposes of this book, medical autonomy refers to the profession's 'legitimated control over the organisation and terms of its own work', while medical dominance refers to 'medicine's authority' over other occupations in the health care division of labour (Elston, 1991:61). Freidson's ([1970a], 1988) early conceptualisation of medical autonomy describes the 'golden age of medicine' during which the profession exercised comprehensive control in all zones of its work. This type of medical autonomy is an ideal which was approximated in the United States from the 1940s to the 1960s (Freidson, 1988). Freidson has since revised and updated his ideas during the 1980s and 1990s as circumstances have changed, particularly in the United States. Dominance theory remains one of the most comprehensive and influential on the professions to date and, moreover, most of the debate since the early 1970s has been in response to his work (Haug, 1973, 1988; Hafferty and Wolinsky, 1991; McKinlay and Arches, 1985, 1986; Rosenthal, 1987). In addition, it provides an invaluable heuristic backdrop against which the nature of autonomy of the medical profession in varying contexts can be appraised, particularly in the absence of baseline information on professions in developing countries.

A clearer portrayal of the nature of medical autonomy in Zimbabwe is made by comparison with the situation existing in Britain and the United States on which most of the theorists on professions have concentrated. Comparison with other developing countries would have been desirable, but there is very little information available on the different dimensions of medical autonomy. Although Johnson's (1973) depiction of professions in post-colonial states is very valuable for this thesis, he does not, for example, delineate the arenas in which the medical profession exercises autonomy.

The specific objectives of the book are to determine the nature and extent of:

1   clinical autonomy among government employed physicians;
2   economic autonomy;
3   regulation of medical education, licensing and medical discipline; and
4   medical dominance.

On the basis of the above, and in the light of existing information on other countries, it is further aimed to arrive at a theoretical characterisation of medical autonomy among government-employed doctors in Zimbabwe.

Rationale for the Book

At a practical policy level, the book will shed light on problems experienced by the Zimbabwe government, with regard to the medical profession including the doctors' strikes of 1988, 1989 and 1994; the persistently high medical turnover which has resulted in acute shortages of medical personnel in government hospitals; and allegations of indiscipline, which include spending more time on private patients and implied neglect of government patients.

A Parliamentary Select Committee appointed in 1992 to investigate the functions of the Health Professions Council revealed that private medical practitioners are poorly regulated by the HPC and other regulatory structures and are, therefore, almost totally unaccountable for their work. The committee concluded that private patients are at risk from possible malpractice by their doctors. This book, which is based on research carried out in the largest government hospital in Zimbabwe, the Parirenyatwa Group of Hospitals, will indicate whether government employed doctors who treat the majority of patients in the country are better regulated than their counterparts in the private sector.

Theoretically, this book is of interest to sociologists of the professions, particularly as much of our understanding of professional autonomy is based on work in developed western countries. Post-colonial states in Africa have evolved quite differently from western developed countries and the political, social, cultural, administrative and economic structures in these countries differ radically from those of developed countries (Bottomore, 1993; Clapham, 1985; Johnson, 1973). Surprisingly, there are still no comprehensive studies analysing the nature of professions in post-colonial states in Africa, even though two decades ago Johnson (1973) chided sociologists for their neglect in this area. Johnson's point is reiterated more recently by Hafferty and Light (1995:148), who charge that 'less well understood, and in many cases unexamined, is the organisation of medical work and the dynamics of professionalism in Third World and developing countries in Africa, Central and South America, Asia and the Pacific Rim'. This lack of studies on developing countries represents a substantial knowledge gap in the Sociology of Professions. Hafferty and Wolinsky (1991) contend that the excessive focus on the situation in the

8

United States has not only 'provincialised' the debate, but has also retarded its advancement, as it now revolves around processes which may be specific to that country. The ultimate aim of this book is to contribute towards filling this gap and the internationalisation of debate.

Johnson (1973) claims that the medical profession in post-colonial states has little autonomy because of its history, the role of the state, and the nature of political relations and social structures in those societies. This book examines the validity of that characterization in the Zimbabwean context. In particular, the book hypothesises that the medical profession in Zimbabwe is essentially different from that of other African countries (as described by Johnson, 1973) because of the nature of both the colonial and post-colonial state and that, for these reasons, it may enjoy more autonomy. Southern Rhodesia, was meant to be a permanent white settler state and an attempt was made by successive colonial governments to create an environment approximating that of the developed western countries for the settlers who, importantly for this book, included medical professionals.

The book is also of interest for comparative analyses of the medical profession in developed countries. Recently, theorists have argued that the medical profession in developed countries no longer has the dominance and autonomy ascribed to it by Freidson (1988), but is losing autonomy through processes allegedly leading to what has variously been described as deprofessionalisation and proletarianisation (Haug, 1973, 1988; McKinlay and Arches, 1985, 1986; McKinlay and Stoeckle, 1986, 1988). Even though the evidence supporting these processes has been seriously challenged for the West (Freidson, 1988, 1989; Navarro, 1988 and others) they still have heuristic and analytical value. This book examines whether such processes are taking place in Zimbabwe and their impact, if any, on medical autonomy.

In western developed countries a process which has been described as 'rolling back the frontiers of the state' (Alaszewski, 1995) is taking place. In Britain, this involves the reduction of the state's role in the provision of social services and increasing privatisation, with the primary intention of curbing public expenditure. At the same time, the state has taken steps to strengthen its hand against professions through the adoption of policies such as managerialism and medical audit (Dent, 1995; Hunter, 1994). Although these policies challenge medical autonomy, the extent of their impact is still not fully clear (Gabe, Kelleher and Williams, 1994). By the late 1980s, Zimbabwe's fiscal crisis had forced it to accept the International Monetary Fund and World Bank prescribed economic structural adjustment programme

(SAP). This entails economic deregulation and privatisation of public institutions, commitment to competition and consumer choice and the reduction and tight control of public spending, particularly on social services. This represents a round-about-turn for a government which had set out to enlarge its role in health care and other public sectors after independence. Not surprisingly, it was forced to abandon or re-examine some of the health policies that it had championed earlier, such as curtailment of the growth of the private medical sector. There has been no assessment of the impact of these processes on medical autonomy in Zimbabwe and this book is able to furnish that information.

Conceptual Framework

Up to the 1960s, most sociologists accepted medicine's depiction of itself as an altruistic profession using its expert knowledge and skills for the benefit of society. Freidson's ([1970b], 1988) professional dominance theory was one of the first and most comprehensive attempts to challenge that view. The theory which was based on an analysis of the Anglo-American situation, describes medicine as an occupation which is distinct from other occupations in the health care sector by virtue of the state-conferred autonomy which it exercises in various aspects of its own work and over the work of others in the sector. The theory gave rise to considerable debate, with some sociologists offering support, for example Zola (1972); Illich (1975), and others maintaining that the medical profession was losing some of its autonomy through processes variously described as deprofessionalisation and proletarianisation (Haug, 1973, 1988; McKinlay and Arches, 1985, 1986; McKinlay and Stoeckle, 1988). The 1990s have seen something of an emerging consensus of opinion among sociologists about the nature of medical autonomy. It is now generally agreed that medical autonomy and dominance are declining due to challenges from inside and outside the health care arena. The most salient of these is from management concerned with regulating the costs and quality of medical care (Freddi and Bjorkman, 1989; Hunter, 1994; Dent, 1995 and Alaszewski, 1995). Other challenges have come from health workers, such as nurses and consumers who are allegedly becoming more demanding and assertive (Witz, 1994). These challenges may bring about a reconfiguration of medical autonomy, but the end result is not clear because the medical profession is fighting back and countering the potential diminution of its autonomy with various strategies, which include wrongly documenting clinical cases in order to obtain higher claims and redirecting patients to outpatient settings where cost-controls are virtually non-existent (Thorpe, 1992, cited in Hunter, 1994).

Freidson (1994) argues that, in analysing the nature of medical autonomy, there is a need to specify the segment of the profession, the level of analysis and the arenas that one is referring to because there is no term that can characterise the level of autonomy of all segments, at every level and in every arena. Some dimensions of medical autonomy, such as clinical and economic autonomy, are exercised by individual physicians, while self-regulation of medical education, licensing and discipline is exercised by the profession as a collectivity. The extent to which physicians exercise autonomy in the various areas of their work varies according to the level of seniority, specialty, occupational role (i.e whether medical bureaucrat, researcher or clinician), employment sector, gender, race, and country of origin (Elston, 1977; Stacey, 1988; Stone, 1980). The medical profession is, in fact, an internally heterogenous collectivity comprising loose amalgamations whose segments pursue different objectives in different ways (Elston, 1977; Freidson, 1994). The extent to which the various segments of the medical profession are impacted by the current challenges to medical dominance and autonomy also varies according to the above variables. Freidson (1994) suggests that the divisions in the profession are getting deeper and eroding the autonomy of some of its sections. Historically, some medical sociologists have failed to appreciate the heterogeneity of the medical profession, often treating doctors either as individuals or as a homogenous group sharing identical beliefs, attitudes and actions. One concern of this book is to underscore the fact that an understanding of the nature of professional autonomy requires a high degree of sensitivity to this issue.

Clinical Autonomy

Clinical autonomy, in the ideal typical form, endows the medical practitioner with the right to determine the entire treatment and management process of the patient, from admission, determination of number and type of diagnostic tests, prescription, surgical or medical procedures to be undertaken and length of stay in hospital. Under these ideal conditions, a physician is responsible only to his or her patient for diagnosis and treatment and only peers can comment on clinical judgement. Any constraints on the practitioner's ability to make these decisions and implement them represent

11

erosion of clinical autonomy, whether they are due to managerial policies aimed at controlling costs and quality of health care or random shortage of resources (Hafferty and Light, 1995).

Haug's (1973) thesis of deprofessionalisation was one of the first to challenge the nature of medical autonomy depicted by Freidson's medical dominance model (Freidson, [1970a], 1988). The thesis claims that medical autonomy is declining due to the diminution of the knowledge gulf between the professional and the general public because of better education than ever before among the public, the effect of the media, widespread public access to computers and the impact of consumer groups (Haug, 1973, 1988). The overall effect of these processes is that clients have become knowledgeable and assertive and want to participate in decision-making concerning their treatment, and are developing the propensity to challenge previously unquestionable decisions made by the practitioner. This undercuts the authority which the doctors have traditionally exercised over clients based on their monopolisation of expertise (Haug, 1973, 1988).

Freidson denies that the knowledge gap has narrowed, arguing that it has in fact widened because medical knowledge is growing at an even faster rate (Freidson, 1989). Contrary to claims by the deprofessionalisation thesis, most patients are not assertive when it comes to the actual encounter with the practitioner who continues to dominate (Freidson, 1989). Evidence to date, however, suggests that a relatively small proportion of dissatisfied consumers complain and an even smaller proportion resort to litigation (Mulcahy and Lloyd Bostock, 1992; Rosenthal, 1987, 1995). Nevertheless, there has been a steep rise in the number of complaints, claims and court cases against the British NHS, which suggests that the public is bolder and more willing to express grievances and concerns (Rosenthal, 1995). However, the rise in frequency of litigation cases in Britain is not confined to the medical profession only, but represents a consumer backlash against all professions.

There is evidence suggesting that the increasing number of female medical practitioners, the critique of the attitudes of the male-dominated medical profession by the feminist movement, and the activities of special interest-groups have gone some way in conscientising women and changing some medical attitudes and practices (Kelleher, 1994). For example, in the treatment of breast cancer patients, medical practitioners used to carry out a biopsy to establish the extent of the cancer invasion while the patient was under anaesthesia and then proceed with surgery, which could include radical mastectomy, without obtaining the patient's consent. This practise has been considerably reduced, largely because of pressure from women's groups, and practitioners have become more sensitive in their treatment of women (Kelleher, 1994). On balance, we can conclude that although some changes have come about as a result of the activities of consumers, their impact on medical autonomy and dominance is far less than envisaged by the deprofessionalisation thesis (Annandale, 1998; Keller, 1994; Rosenthal, 1987).

The deprofessionalisation thesis also claims that computer technology threatens medical autonomy as is becoming evident in Britain where computers are being utilised in the development of coding schemes. In the United States, they are employed in the storing and retrieving of clinical protocols and diagnostic related groups (DRGs) used as bench marks for professional practice (Dohler, 1989; Haug, 1988; Light, 1988). The deprofessionalisation hypothesis, like the dominance theory which it hopes to supplant is limited to an analysis of the Anglo-American context. Consequently, its relevance to analysing the state of medical autonomy in developing countries appears limited since it presupposes the existence of well educated consumers who have easy access to computers.

Most sociologists now agree that there is an erosion of clinical autonomy largely from governments and other health providers concerned with regulating rising costs and the quality of medical care, but they are not agreed on the end result of the process. Clinical autonomy is no longer sacrosanct and is under threat from health providers intent on containing health costs, an estimated 80 per cent of which are incurred by medical decisions (Dohler, 1989). In the United States, the process started in the 1960s with the public's concern over the ethicality and protection of the rights of 'human subjects' (Freidson, 1989). Accordingly, methods used in research programmes involving human beings had to be reviewed for technical propriety and moral acceptability whenever funded by the federal government. After the introduction of Medicare and Medicaid, all medical decisions concerning hospitalisation and length of stay of patients under these schemes were reviewed by a formal review committee (Freidson, 1989). Medical effectiveness research aimed at establishing better clinical protocols threatens to further limit clinical discretion, particularly if administered by non-medical managers, even if the actual research is carried out by medical professionals (Hafferty and Light, 1995).

In Britain, before the advent of the recent health reforms which started in 1979, the government had overall financial control, but doctors bore the main burden of rationing health care. For example, it was the medical profession which decided who could have access to the limited number of kidney machines available in the country (Klein, 1989; Harrison and Pollitt, 1994). This arrangement has been eroded by the 1990s reforms in the health sector, especially the introduction of general practitioner fund-holding and medical audit. The medical profession is attempting to reduce these challenges to clinical autonomy by assuming the management positions themselves to ensure that reforms are not implemented by non-medical people (Hunter, 1994). In spite of the constraints brought about by the reforms in the health sector, the British medical profession continues to exercise more clinical autonomy than their American counterparts who have had more stringent performance and cost monitoring systems for much longer (Dohler, 1989; Harrison and Schulz, 1989; Hunter, 1994).

The erosion of clinical autonomy has been enhanced by the change in the role of managers, who are no longer merely advisory, but are now becoming more directive and definitive. Where previously practitioners could pay little attention to their advice, this is no longer the case (Freidson, 1985). But, as pointed out earlier, some practitioners in the United States avoid cost and quality control measures which impinge on their clinical and economic autonomy by carrying out more medical work in their private surgeries where there is little managerial regulation. The DRG programmes have also been rendered less effective by practitioners who provide inadequate information on diagnoses, wrongly coding the conditions treated and generally being uncooperative in order to earn more money and minimise the erosion of their clinical and economic autonomy (Hunter, 1994).

The threat of litigation for malpractice threatens clinical autonomy, as medical practitioners in the United States become more careful and cover themselves from possible allegations of malpractice by engaging in defensive medicine. They increase the number of medical procedures that they carry out in order to protect themselves, which in turn pushes up medical costs while at the same time increasing the income of medical professionals (Light, 1993). The conclusion from the available evidence suggests that the battery of clinical control programmes erode the clinical discretion of individual practitioners but as will be discussed below, the dominant position of the medical profession in the health care division of labour remains underpinned by licensing laws (Bjorkman, 1989; Freidson, 1989; Larkin, 1993; Light, 1991).

Comprehensive economic autonomy gives the medical practitioner the right to decide: their type of employment, whether solo fee-for-service, group practice or salaried employment in bureaucratic organisations; type of remuneration; location of employment; time of work; and choice of client. Advocates of the proletarianisation thesis claim that the medical profession is undergoing a transformation and losing control of some of the prerogatives that it formerly enjoyed as a result of increasing employment in bureaucratic organisations (McKinlay and Arches, 1985, 1986; McKinlay and Stoeckle, 1986, 1988; Oppenheimer, 1973). The essential aspect of the proletarianisation process is the progressive stripping of the profession's control over a number of prerogatives such as control of entry to the profession, training, terms and content of work and rate of remuneration (McKinlay and Arches, 1985). These are increasingly falling under the control of private and public bureaucrats who, as trustees of organisational resources regulate and control the activities of professionals in an effort to reduce costs (Oppenheimer, 1973). The programmes are devised for the benefit of the organisation and not for the profession and therefore represent a challenge to medical autonomy, regardless of who administers them (Hafferty and Light, 1995). Wolinsky (1988:43) however, asserts that medical managers continue to identify with the profession, unless they 'fully and completely divest themselves of all actual medical practise'.

The notion that salaried employment leads to proletarianisation has been rejected by many scholars (cf. Freidson, 1988, 1989; Elston, 1991; Navarro, 1988; Rosenthal, 1987). In fact, 'employment status does not in and of itself mean a loss of economic independence. If one's position in the labour market is strong, one can specify the terms and conditions of one's employment granting little power to the employer' (Freidson, 1989:187). Contrary to common belief, self-employed professionals are not as autonomous as they appear because they are 'at the mercy of consumer's terms and conditions and an unpredictable market' (Freidson, 1989:187). Evidence in support of this comes from British physicians who lost the right to determine their remuneration from patients in 1949, but were sheltered from the economic vulnerability of solo fee-for-service practice (Elston, 1991; Johnson, 1995). Consultants are not only assured of a stable income from the NHS, but they also retain the right to practise privately, which gives them considerable economic autonomy. However, the British medical profession has not been able to dictate its own terms of remuneration from the state, hence the long history of pay disputes since the inception of the NHS (Elston, 1991). But, in comparison with other health occupations, physicians have more power in pay negotiations.

Physicians in the United States enjoy more economic autonomy than their British counterparts who have less opportunities for practising privately because the NHS is still the main provider of health care. In addition, United States physicians have in the past been able to increase their income by carrying out unnecessary and costly procedures. Such opportunities are declining with the increasing effectiveness of management initiated cost controls and peer review programmes, but to get round these, medical professionals are investing heavily in their own buildings and equipment (Light, 1993).

The contention that specialisation leads to declining incomes, as claimed by proletarianisation advocates, although initially refuted by Light and Levine (1988), appears imminent in the United States due to the looming over-supply of specialists. This raises the danger of intra-professional clashes as specialists encroach on the turf of general practitioners because of a shortage of demand for specialist services (Light, 1993). Each specialty forms its own representative body and the proliferation of different specialty bodies raises the potential of intra-professional competition for prestige and resources (Freidson, 1988; Light, 1993). For example, sub-specialties in America have been making attempts to legally exclude family practitioners from carrying out certain procedures (Light, 1993).

Some theorists have contended that the economic autonomy and dominance of the medical profession are under threat from other workers in the health care division of labour and from alternative health practitioners. The nursing profession in Britain, for example, embarked on Project 2000 with the aim of enhancing its occupational status and creating a niche for itself distinct from medicine with but these efforts are likely to result in the restratification of the profession, as elite members take duties previously performed by the general practitioners, while the situation of the majority remains unchanged (Witz, 1994). In addition, Witz (1994) contends that caring, which nursing is declaring as its own, is commonly identified with women's work, which has always had a low status. Even though these efforts represent a challenge to medical dominance, nurses continue to operate in areas determined for them by the medical profession and underpinned by licensing and credentialing laws (Hugman, 1992; Larkin, 1983, 1995).

Challenges to medical dominance from alternative health practitioners have come about partly as a result of the public's disillusionment with the ineffectiveness of biomedicine in curing degenerative chronic diseases and what are seen as its dehumanising effects (Gabe, Kelleher and Williams, 1994). Consequently, therapies that were previously excluded from the NHS, such as osteopathy, homeopathy and acupuncture, and more recently, reflexology and aromatherapy, are gaining in popularity (Saks, 1995). Saks (1994) concludes that alternative therapies do not seriously threaten medical dominance and hence its privileged economic position while Larkin (1995) sees their incorporation into the NHS as an extension of the medico-bureaucratic alliance rather than a threat to the dominance of the medical profession.

Johnson (1973), who looked at professions in post-colonial states, contends that the medical profession has very little autonomy because of the social structures and power relations which exist in those societies. The difference is largely attributed to the nature of the relationship between the state and the professions and their historical development under colonialism. Some weak rudiments of professionalism may appear in post-colonial states due to the presence of Western expatriate professionals and of indigenous professionals trained in developed countries. Patronage, which is pervasive in these societies, weakens the role of professional associations and it is inconceivable, that 'successful private practise could be achieved and maintained without official support or at least tacit agreement of the authorities' (Johnson, 1973:299). In any case, the opportunities for practising private medicine are very small because there is no large heterogenous group of middle class citizens who can afford to pay for private medical care. Consequently, the medical profession in post-colonial states has very little economic autonomy (Johnson, 1973). Johnson's observations were made only a few years after the independence of most of the African countries, and what may have obtained then may not be the case over twenty years later, particularly after the wave of democratic and multi-party politics which swept the African continent in the late 1980s and early 1990s. In addition, most post-colonial states have adopted the IMF and World Bank-enforced liberalisation policies as part of economic structural adjustment programmes. As we will see later in this chapter and in Chapter 3, Zimbabwe's colonial history differs somewhat from that of these other countries and it is quite likely that the nature of economic autonomy enjoyed by the physicians may differ from that portrayed by Johnson (1973).

The medical profession in Britain and the United States secured the right to exercise self-regulation in the areas of education, licensing and discipline in the nineteenth century. Collective autonomy gives the medical profession the right to control entry to the profession, determine the curriculum, judge the competence of its members and, consequently, determine those who have deviated from the laid down expectations of professional and clinical conduct and deserve disciplinary action. In the last twenty years, an increasingly sceptical and assertive public has expressed dissatisfaction with the quality of medical care and the lack of adequate monitoring and regulation of doctors, particularly since the medical profession in most societies has failed to ensure the continued competence of its members (Rosenthal, 1987; Stacey, 1992). The American Medical Association (AMA) has attempted to address that issue by providing continuing education for its members, sponsoring refresher courses and awarding of research grants (Freidson, 1988). The GMC, on the other hand, has no mechanisms to ensure that doctors keep up with developments in their area and for ensuring improvement for those who display deficient professional performance (Rosenthal, 1995).

The public's frustration with the way the profession monitors and disciplines its members has partly promoted a litigious tendency among Americans. Increasingly, the medical profession in both the United States and Britain is moving towards more formal methods of evaluating each other's clinical performance rather than relying almost entirely on the informal but largely ineffective methods which they have traditionally depended on. Stacey (1992) points out that the British General Medical Council (GMC) has reluctantly accepted the need for other practitioners to assess colleagues' clinical performance and report on those suspected of committing serious professional misconduct. Up to 1992, deprecation of colleague's 'professional skill, knowledge, qualifications or services' could raise questions of serious professional misconduct, according to the GMC guidelines for norms of professional behaviour, but this has since been changed to enable doctors to judge and report on colleague's clinical competence (cited in Rosenthal, 1995:5). The reluctant and rather belated acceptance of medical audit and peer review by the British medical profession is part of this shift from informal to more formal mechanisms of self-regulation. In the mid-1990s, the GMC is considering accepting complaints dealing with professional competence as one of its disciplinary responsibilities (Rosenthal, 1995). In the United States, the introduction of informer laws which make it mandatory for physicians to report on colleagues guilty of malpractice has gone some way in reducing the profession's tendency of protecting and not testifying against each other in courts of law (Freidson, 1989).

Johnson (1973) argues that the medical profession in post-colonial states does not have strong professional associations to fight for self-regulation in education, registration and discipline like their counterparts in developed western countries such as Britain and the United States. These are either the responsibility of a state department or other institutions responsible to the state. At most, the professional associations in post-colonial states fight to have a medical education syllabus which is acceptable to the British General Medical Council and other overseas medical associations. Similarly, the associations have not developed an independent code of ethics, but have merely duplicated the British one (Johnson, 1973). Understandably, the structures for enforcement of discipline are weak.

The first aim of the above discussion of the three dimensions of medical autonomy was to provide a general introductory background of the concepts which guided analysis of the empirical findings on Zimbabwe presented in the chapters which follow. Our theoretical review showed that the current theories of professions are ethnocentric in nature, all of them being essentially premised on the Anglo-American medical experience. Dominance theory as we noted earlier describes the 'golden era' which was a specific historically bound phenomenon. Deprofessionalisation and proletarianisation hypotheses which attempt to replace dominance theory are no better in this respect as they too focus on changes taking place in the United States. Accordingly, the second aim was to remind ourselves of the present state of knowledge on medical autonomy and to highlight the gaps in our knowledge on the nature of medical autonomy in post-colonial and developing countries which this book hopes to fill.

We have seen that medical autonomy is state-conferred status but it is important to appreciate that the degree to which a profession exercises it varies according to the nature and role of the state in medical care in the given society (Frenk and Durans-Arenas, 1993; Freidson, 1988; Garpenby, 1989; Johnson, 1972). Many studies which have examined the degree of autonomy exercised by the medical profession in different societies have amply demonstrated that this varies widely even among the different western developed capitalist countries (Dohler, 1989; Freddi and Bjorkman, 1989; Garpenby, 1989; Harrison and Schulz, 1989; Rosenthal, 1987, 1988, 1995).

For example, even though the history of professionalisation of medicine in the United States and Britain is comparable, the professions exercise different degrees of medical autonomy essentially because of the nature of the state (Freidson, 1988; Starr, 1983). Similarly, although doctors in both Britain and Sweden work in public systems and are salaried, the degree of professional autonomy and self-regulation exercised by doctors in the two countries differs considerably (Garpenby, 1989; Rosenthal, 1987, 1988, 1995). Frenk and Durans-Arenas (1993) emphasize that the state is the most influential actor determining the relative strength of the medical profession and other groups in society. Below we examine the nature of the Zimbabwean state in order to understand the administrative, political, economic, cultural and social context in which health policies are formulated and implemented and some of the underlying assumptions and interests. This is crucial, given that most commentators on the Zimbabwe state maintain that most post-colonial government policies are fettered by inherited and other objective constraints (Loewenson, 1988, 1990; Mandaza, 1987; Stoneman, 1988; Wood, 1987).

The Zimbabwean State

This section briefly reviews some of the important characteristics of post-colonial states before analysing the Zimbabwe state in terms of: its political heritage; administrative structures; the nature of its economy; the social development agenda; and its relationship with the civil society.

We follow Frenk and Durans-Arenas's (1993) narrow definition of the state as a set of institutions comprising the legislature, executive, judiciary, police and armed forces which exercise public authority and power. Its most important attribute, following Weber (1978), is that it has political domination in addition to attaining the legitimate use of force within a given territory (Abercrombie, Hill and Turner, 1988). Government on the other hand, refers to 'specific occupants of office' involved in decision making at a particular time (Chazan et al, 1992).

The question of whether the post-colonial state should be viewed as different from developed states has been amply and convincingly answered in the affirmative by a number of theorists who argue that developing countries have unique features which are distinct from those of developed countries because of their history, level of economic and industrial development, political, social and cultural traditions (Bottomore, 1992;

20

Chazan *et al*, 1992; Clapham, 1985; Holder-Williams, 1984; Tordoff, 1984). These theorists have generally characterised the post-colonial state as centralised, authoritarian and impermeable (Clapham, 1985; Chazan *et al*, 1992). The post-colonial state, which is essentially a continuation of its predecessor is based on rational-legal principles, while the cultural beliefs, attitudes and practices of its people are largely those of pre-industrial societies in which loyalty to one's kin group is of primary social value and where patrimonialism pervades both the political and administrative structures. Not surprisingly, most of these societies have had problems working according to rational-legal bureaucratic principles.

Even though most post-colonial states espoused ideologies which were essentially different from those of the colonial powers, no logistic and theoretical considerations were given for transformation of the economy in accordance with the ideologies (Mandaza, 1986). Although post-colonial states attained political independence, they remain extremely constrained by their subordinate and dependent position in the international economic system to which they were linked through colonialism and later by their relationship with international finance institutions such as the World Bank and the International Monetary Fund (Bottomore, 1992; Clapham, 1985). Hodder-Williams (1984) contends that in the absence of an indigenous private sector and entrenched pressure groups, the post-colonial state is a monopolistic state, with multinational corporations and international aid agencies as the only countervailing sources of power.

Colonial Origins

Rhodesia (now Zimbabwe) was colonised by a British multinational corporation, the British South Africa Company, in 1890 (see Figure 1.1) for geographical location). Prior to colonisation, the territory now known as Zimbabwe was inhabited by the Shona and the Ndebele, now constituting about 78 and 19 per cent respectively, who were engaged in agriculture and mining and traded successfully with the Portuguese in the territory now known as Mozambique (Palmer, 1979). Unlike the situation in most other colonies, the immigrants to Rhodesia were not employees of the British colonial office, but were settlers who intended to make the colony their home. As one former governor aptly put it, 'in the British colonies, people go home every thirty months, in Rhodesia, they go home every night' (cited in Gelfand, 1976:9).

21

Africans were systematically dispossessed of fertile land to give to settlers and at the same time create a reservoir of labourers to work in the white agricultural, mining, manufacturing and domestic sectors (Van Onselen, 1976). One of the most tragic results of colonial land policies was that formerly self-sufficient indigenous people were consciously and systematically transformed into cheap wage labourers and landless or impoverished subsistence farmers through successive laws such as the Land Apportionment Act (1930) and successive Maize Control acts (Stoneman and Cliffe, 1989). This had far reaching results, including a general decline in the health status of the indigenous population, as we will see in Chapter 3.

In 1923, the settlers opted for the status of 'responsible government' under the British and in 1953, the colony joined two other central African states, Northern Rhodesia (Zambia) and Nyasaland (Malawi) to form the Federation of Rhodesia and Nyasaland, which broke up ten years later in 1963 due to increased demands for independence by Nyasaland and Northern Rhodesia. When the two latter countries were granted independence, most of the settlers from these countries migrated to Southern Rhodesia which already had a large settler population. The settlers in Rhodesia who were opposed to majority rule declared unilateral independence (UDI) from Britain in 1965 and changed the country's name to Rhodesia. The period following UDI was marked by consolidation of the whites' economic and political position and increased racial discrimination. The settler government tried and succeeded in forging unity and support for itself by creating 'socialism for the whites' in which all the settlers were shielded from competition with Africans, and consequently, enjoyed an extraordinarily high standard of living (Herbst, 1990:22). At the same time, erosion of African economic capacity was contrived through forced removals from fertile land; reservation of skilled, professional and managerial jobs in both industry and the civil service for the white community; and denial of the right and financial resources to engage in viable entrepreneurial activity in urban areas (Stoneman and Cliff, 1989). Stoneman (1988:43) argues that Rhodesian society was one of the most unequal in the world, with the average white earnings more than ten times those of blacks in formal employment. For example, in 1980, of the 10,570 tenured posts in the civil service, blacks occupied 3,368 with none holding a position higher than senior administrative officer (*Herald*, 18 April, 1985). The whites, comprising 3 per cent of the country's population, owned two thirds of the best land; and nearly all of the mining and industrial rights. The Rhodesian state, which was founded by a multinational corporation, had a special

Figure 1.1   Geographical Location of Zimbabwe

ZIMBABWE

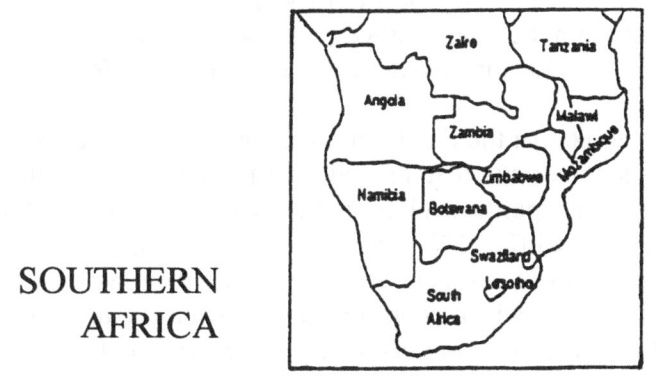

SOUTHERN
AFRICA

relationship with both local and international capital, which it provided with infrastructure and subsidy support necessary for its survival (Herbst, 1990).

Black nationalists' opposition to the settlers' racial, repressive and inequitable policies which denied them political rights and gave rise to serious economic deprivation, found expression in a ten year armed struggle against the colonial state starting in the late 1960s. The main issue on which the guerillas agreed and for which they received support from the indigenous population, was the promise that they would take back the expropriated land and redistribute it to the indigenous population. The guerilla war was led by two main nationalist parties, the Zimbabwe African National Union (ZANU) and the Zimbabwe African People's Union (ZAPU), which fought from military bases in Mozambique and Zambia, respectively. Thousands of young blacks left Rhodesia to train as guerilla fighters in Mozambique, China, Yugoslavia, Cuba, Tanzania and North Korea and on their return as guerilla fighters, they attacked strategic installations like oil storage tanks, electricity and bridges and generally disrupted large-scale farming, forcing some white farmers to abandon their farms. It is estimated that between twenty and thirty thousand lives were lost during the ten years of war (Stoneman and Cliffe, 1989). By the late 1970s, the settler government was experiencing serious military and economic difficulties and white emigration to South Africa, Britain, Australia and New Zealand was escalating.

In 1978, the settler government brokered an internal settlement with black nationalists inside Rhodesia and installed a puppet interim government led by Bishop Muzorewa and the country was renamed Zimbabwe-Rhodesia. Independent African states refused to recognise Zimbabwe-Rhodesia and the liberation movements continued to fight the interim government, which lasted slightly over a year. Meanwhile, increasing apprehension on the part of the United States and British governments that an in-coming black government would lean towards the Soviet sphere of influence motivated them to put pressure on the interim government and former settler rulers to negotiate with the nationalist movements at Lancaster House in 1979 (Herbst, 1990).

Analysts agree that the timely intervention by the United States and Britain was intended to ensure that the military superiority of the nationalists was not translated into political clout at the negotiating table (Mandaza, 1986; Stoneman and Cliffe, 1989; Herbst, 1990). Both the British and United States governments wanted to ensure that there was no radical transformation of society which could threaten their economic interests, as most of the multinational corporations in the country were either of British,

24

United States or South African origin. The then United States representative to the United Nations aptly summed up his country's intentions, 'the US has but one option, and that is neo-colonialism' (quoted in Stoneman and Cliffe, 1989:29).

Lancaster House Constitution

The Lancaster House constitution, which could practically not be amended for the first ten years of independence, was intended to entrench the existing legal, administrative and socio-economic institutions. The terms of the Lancaster House Constitution gave the black nationalists political power, but ensured that whites retained economic power (Mandaza, 1986). The brokers of the independence settlement fought for the preservation of the state machinery, allegedly to 'maintain high standards' and inspire the 'confidence' of both the settlers and the international community in the new state (Mandaza, 1986:34).

One of the lynch pins of the Lancaster House Constitution was the Bill of Rights, which safeguarded capitalism and its institutional pillars. It stated, among other things, that regardless of how land and mining rights were originally obtained, they could only change hands on a 'willing seller, willing buyer' basis (Stoneman, 1988:45). Any government purchase of privately owned capital assets was to be made in foreign currency, based on the going market prices and paid for immediately. Mozambique and Zambia were pressurised by the United States and British governments, on whom they depended for economic aid, to persuade the Zimbabwean nationalists to accept the Lancaster House Constitution. The nationalists were duly informed that if they rejected it, they could no longer locate their bases in Mozambique and both ZANU and ZAPU which had hoped to secure outright victory against the Rhodesian army, had no option but to accept the unfavourable Constitution. The British government made the Constitution slightly more acceptable for the nationalists by promising a massive grant for purchasing land for redistribution but later only gave fifty million pounds as a 'development fund' (Stoneman and Cliffe, 1989:33).

The Constitution made it impossible for the post-colonial government to obtain land on the basis of justice or need and this effectively meant that unless government could obtain large amounts of foreign currency for this purpose, the whites were going to continue to own over 50 per cent of the economy, including most of the fertile land and most of the mining and manufacturing sectors (Stoneman, 1988). The cash-strapped

Zimbabwean government was unable to effectively fulfil its most important election promises, redistribution of land and eradication of landlessness and overcrowding in the rural areas.

Post-independence Administrative Structures and Practices

As explained above, the structure of Zimbabwean society as determined at Lancaster House differed considerably from other African countries at the time of their independence. Mandaza (1986:50) argues that Zimbabwe was more than just a neo-colonial state, being 'born fettered and historically constrained by ... imperialism'. Most African countries which attained independence before Zimbabwe succeeded weak colonial administrations with scant institutional structures intended for the small white colonial administration which serviced the colony. Post-colonial governments in these countries, therefore, had the opportunity to create their own administrative structures and policy-making apparatus.

In addition, other African countries had more autonomy in the creation of state institutions because the colonial powers were not as concerned about what happened after independence as they were in the case of Zimbabwe where they had strong economic interests and kith and kin to protect (Mandaza, 1986). For example, in Zambia, the colonial administration was very small and concerned, above all, with facilitating the exploitation of mineral wealth and maintenance of law and order. The post-independence Zambian government was therefore able to create most of its own state institutions where there had been virtually none before.

In the case of Zimbabwe, there had been a strong government with entrenched institutions and practices whose survival the Lancaster House Constitution had secured. Traditions of the civil service based on the rational-legal principle, such as anonymity, political neutrality, impartiality, separation of public office from the person, and security of tenure were to be guaranteed by the constitution. The inherited colonial bureaucratic machinery was massive, but very effective, compared to other African countries and was capable of running the civil service and regulating the economy largely through a corporatist network (Herbst, 1990; Stoneman and Cliffe, 1989).

The ruling party, ZANU, which had witnessed first hand the administrative and economic chaos that ensued in Mozambique when the Portuguese left that country on the eve of independence, adopted a policy of reconciliation in order to reassure the whites and convince them to remain in the country. This essentially meant that the new government was not going to seek revenge on the former rulers and the settlers for what had gone on before independence and in return, it was hoped that the settlers would accept the new political order and remain in the country. Another reason why the new government adopted reconciliation was to appease hostile South Africa, which seriously considered invading Zimbabwe soon after independence because it did not want a successful socialist-oriented country on its doorstep (Hanlon, 1988).

Due to the racist practices of the colonial government, all the black members of the new cabinet had no previous government experience, and had to rely on experienced white civil servants to formulate and implement policies in the first few years. Bratton (1981 cited in Herbst, 1990:31) aptly sums up the situation in which the new government found itself:

> At independence, the ZANU (PF) leadership constituted a thin veneer atop a largely untransformed state apparatus. The Cabinet found itself in a fragile position because institutions wholly or partly controlled by groups of dubious loyalty were interposed between the leadership and its popular base.

In 1984, the ruling party, ZANU (PF) declared its supremacy over the government and the Political Bureau (Politburo), which is the supreme body of the ruling party, comprising a small group of the most senior party members, including some ministers, became the main policy-making body, responsible for supervising the implementation of government policies and the general performance of government (Stoneman and Cliffe, 1989). A number of government ministers, including the current Minister of Health, are not members of this policy-making body and, therefore, do not take part in the formulation of policies for their ministries, nor can they directly defend the performance of their ministries. Since the present Minister of Health does not sit in the policy-making body, he learns about decisions relating to his ministry from the Secretary for Health in the Political Bureau, who also heads his own government ministry.

As the basic tenets of the government's policies in most ministries are now in place, the Political Bureau and the cabinet largely ratify policies initiated from the ministries. For example, the Ministry of Health was essentially implementing the policies outlined by the first Minister of Health in 1980 without much alteration up to 1990 when the government adopted the Structural Adjustment Program (SAP) proposed by international donor agencies. More recently, it was the Political Bureau which insisted that the minimum salary for those paying hospital fees should be raised from Z$150 to Z$400 per month so that more families could be exempted from paying fees.

Soon after independence, the government embarked on an Africanisation process in which suitably qualified but inexperienced blacks were hired to government posts, while elderly whites were offered early retirement packages. By 1983, most of the key civil service posts, from assistant to permanent secretary, were occupied by blacks, most of whom were technocrats rather than political stalwarts. Herbst (1990) argues that the process of Africanisation did not necessarily guarantee the new political leaders state control, particularly since they had to rely on civil servants who were sometimes accused of 'hijacking' government policies and forming an 'invisible cabinet'. A former senior civil servant in the Ministry of Health explained to me in interview that when policies he did not agree with were proposed, he engaged delaying tactics to ensure that they were not adopted. On the suggested policy of phasing out private medicine, his department calculated the financial implications of that policy and then informed the Ministry of Finance and Economic Development that, in the absence of a private medical sector, the Ministry of Health would need three times its current budget to meet everyone's health care needs. The Minister of Finance advised cabinet on the folly of such a policy and the cabinet decided to leave the private sector intact. The differences in ideological orientation in the ranks of the political and administrative elite went some way in undermining the proposed health care agenda.

The State and the Economy

Zimbabwe inherited one of the strongest economies in Southern Africa, mostly comprising agriculture, mining and manufacturing, most of which is privately owned, 75 per cent of it by foreign transnational companies such as Lonrho, Anglo-American and Unilever. The economic sector had enjoyed very close relations with the colonial state, maintained through a corporatist 'old boy' network, as state officials and the owners of capital shared the same racial, cultural and ideological heritage (Herbst, 1990; Stoneman, 1981). The relationship which existed between the post-colonial state and the private economic sector was hostile, with the state resenting the private sector which had helped sustain the colonial regime and remained exclusively white and largely foreign owned. The private sector was opposed to the government's professed socialism which discouraged foreign investment, gave workers 'too many rights' and created an ambitious social services programme which raised taxation levels. However, in spite of its socialist rhetoric, the government relied on the private sector for revenue and therefore had to create an enabling environment.

Sticking to the spirit of reconciliation meant abandonment of the socialist political agenda, since there could not be any radical redistribution of land and other private economic assets without violating it. Accordingly, the then Prime Minister Robert Mugabe, announced soon after independence that the new government accepted the reality of capitalism (Sibanda, 1988). All these factors, but especially the terms of the Lancaster House Constitution, ensured that the private sector became a countervailing force against the implementation of the state's socialist principles. The private economic sector had strong external allies to protect it against any hostile action, such as nationalisation by the government, and could therefore stand in opposition to government without fear of being victimised in any way. Not surprisingly, the state has had difficulty getting the private sector to play the game according to its rules (Nyaruwata, 1988).

In its policies towards workers, the state was concerned with introducing a minimum wage for lowly paid workers and improving industrial relations (Davies, 1988). Although it introduced a new Labour Relations Act which gave workers some rights in the work place, the grievance settling procedure remained essentially the same as the colonial one which was cumbersome and frustrating (Sachikonye, 1987). Even the management style and industrial relations in government-owned corporations were no more socialist than those of foreign owned companies (Mutizwa-Mangiza, 1988). This confirmed the conclusions of many social analysts who argue that there exists a gap between political rhetoric and what exists on the ground in Zimbabwe (Sibanda, 1988; Nyaruwata, 1988; Stoneman, 1988). In fact, the state further constrained its options for socialist transformation by appealing to the international donor countries and agencies to support its social development programmes (Nyaruwata, 1988; Mandaza, 1986; Chakaodza, 1993).

The government's ambitious social welfare programme could not be met with internal revenue, so it sought foreign aid for implementation. The Zimbabwe government believed that it could mobilise foreign capital to fulfil popular expectations but social analysts have questioned its naivety in expecting capitalist donor countries and agencies to fund its socialist programmes (Mandaza, 1986; Stoneman, 1988). The private economic sector, comprising local and multinational corporations controlling mining, manufacturing and large-scale agriculture in Zimbabwe counted donor agencies and countries as their strongest bulwark against hostile activities of the state. Thus donor countries and agencies became an influential countervailing force which the state had to contend with in both its internal and external policies. The options of the state have dwindled as the countervailing power of international finance institutions has grown, and as we will see in chapters 5 and 6, this has had a significant impact on health care provision and medical autonomy.

The government's heavy development programme resulted in deficits in both the internal budget and external payments, further steeping the country into debt and the dictates of foreign donors. From a state of being under-borrowed in 1981, with a debt estimated at 16 per cent of GDP, this rose to 53 per cent by 1984 (Stoneman, 1988). By 1987, the government had accepted that its economic policies did not enable servicing of its foreign debt and maintenance of its ambitious social development programme (Hawkins, 1993). In 1990, the government accepted an IMF/World Bank-initiated Structural Adjustment Programme which compelled it to: reduce public sector spending on education, health and housing; reduce public sector employment; remove subsidies; privatise public corporations and the provision of public services; deregulate labour relations; remove administrative controls and generally liberalise the economy (Chakaodza, 1993). In essence, the state was being forced by the donor countries and aid agencies to reverse its social development programmes which mostly benefitted the poor majority. As we have seen earlier in this chapter, some of the health policies which the government espoused had the potential of reducing medical autonomy but, as we will note in Chapters 5 and 6, some of these were abandoned while others were amended because of the opposition of the medical profession, supported by both local and international finance agencies. These external factors which are so salient in policy-making in developing countries are of little or no significance to developed Western countries and the autonomy of their medical professions.

The Post-independence Social Development Agenda

Formulation and implementation of the government's espoused socialist policies were seriously constrained by existing socio-economic and legal realities. Mandaza (1986) describes post-colonial Zimbabwe as a schizophrenic state attempting to formulate and implement radical developmental policies to benefit the majority of the population in the face of economic and political pressure from donor countries and finance institutions which attempt to ensure that those aspirations are not met. He argues that the inevitable contradictions affect every institution of the post-colonial state.

Davies (1988) examines the country's achievements in socio-economic development, including health and education, from 1980 to 1988 and concludes that the achievements, though impressive in some areas, are reformist and compatible with a welfare capitalist rather than socialist economy. The Labour Relations Act passed in 1985, gave black workers some rights in the work place and made it difficult for employers to sack them without the permission of the Ministry of Labour, Manpower and Social Services. There was also some land redistribution to meet the needs of some of the landless people, but unfortunately, most of the beneficiaries were resettled in the less desirable agro-ecological regions of the country. Mandaza (1986) and Davies (1988) point out that such expansion occurred in most post-colonial African states almost regardless of their professed political ideology. Several attempts have been made to explain why there is a gap between most of the government's proposed plans and what was happening on the ground. Some have attributed this to lack of clear socialist development plans because the ruling party leadership, which was essentially a mixed bag of radical marxists, old guard militant nationalists, politically neutral technocrats, and petty bourgeois professionals and academics had no ideological consensus (Mandaza, 1987, 1991; Stoneman, 1988; Stoneman and Cliffe, 1989).

The absence of a clearly articulated development plan left room for conflicts between the different factions in the national leadership, particularly between the socialists and the technocratic element in the cabinet, but more importantly, in the way in which the broad policies could be interpreted by the technocratic civil servants who had to formulate specific policies and implement them. The example involving a former senior servant in the Ministry of Health discussed earlier is a case in point. Such occurrences gave the nation the impression that the cabinet was divided and undecided, leaving it open to exploitation by opposed interests.

State-society Relations

As discussed earlier, the Zimbabwean state never became as dominant and centralised as other African states because of the Lancaster House constitution as well as opposition from the relatively strong private economic

31

sector, the international community, and civil groups within Zimbabwean society. Other factors such as patrimonialism, corruption and impermeability did begin to emerge and, by the late 1980s, the Zimbabwean public had become cynical of the political leadership and its policies. Armed with evidence of political corruption and unresponsiveness to public demands in the government leadership, the public refused to give the government the chance to further insulate itself by establishing one party state.

Zimbabwean society, familiar with the legacy of economic stagnation, corruption and political intransigency bequeathed on other African states by the one party system, made its opposition quite clear. One writer captured the public's feelings when he wrote an article entitled, 'Should Zimbabwe be going where others are coming from?' (Sithole, 1991). An opposition party was even formed with most of its support based on opposition to political corruption and rejection of a one party state. The public's apathy in the 1990 elections, in which the one party system issue was on the ruling party's election manifesto, went some way in convincing the ruling party to abandon the idea of imposing the system against the people's will and in 1990, the President announced that his party was shelving the idea.

The public was worried that the political leadership would use the one party state to further its own position and interests, as signs of political degeneracy and complacency had already begun to manifest themselves. In 1984, the then Prime Minister (now Executive President) publicly condemned some of his ministers and senior civil servants for deceiving the public and accumulating private property. He asked them 'to quit or relinquish their property' (*Herald*, 16 August, 1984, cited in Sibanda, 1988, 262). There were public demonstrations by women and university students protesting the corruption and capitalist activities of some ministers. Revelations of political corruption and accumulation of personal wealth using public office highlighted the duplicity of the political leadership which continued to proclaim its intention of transforming the country's economy to socialism. The public was especially wary in view of the party's inability to control its own acquisitive members.

In 1984, the then Secretary-General of the ruling party, Maurice Nyagumbo, explained to the nation that the party had failed to enforce a leadership code among the party's leadership. The leadership code prohibited senior party and government officials from owning businesses; receiving more than one salary; and serving as directors of private firms or business organised for profit. Acceptance of private accumulation by the party leadership meant that government could not prohibit other members of society from accumulating personal wealth and this also opened the possibility for government officials and other members of the public to use their offices for personal gain. There was a very real danger that corruption was going to become a pervasive feature of Zimbabwean society, as the state President aptly put it, 'if gold rusts, what will iron do?' (cited in Sithole, 1991:77). Mandaza (1991) asks why leaders alone were expected to conform in a society in which whites and blacks in the private sector were allowed to amass wealth and were not criticised for it?

The first public evidence of corruption by senior political leaders was revealed by the media in 1987 in what became known as the 'Willowgate Scandal' (Stoneman and Cliffe, 1989). A number of senior government officials used their public positions to acquire cars from the Willowvale Motor Company (at a time when there was a severe shortage of cars on the market) and then sold them above the government stipulated prices. The Sandura Commission (1987), appointed by the President to investigate the matter, revealed that a number of ministers and other senior government officials had taken part in car racketeering. When the President asked the law to take its course, the public hailed the public revelations of the Commission's findings and the President's non-interference as evidence of the government's desire to maintain transparency and public accountability.

Five ministers were found guilty in the court of law and fined, and subsequently resigned from their government posts and the Secretary-General of the party who had also been implicated, committed suicide while the one minister who was sent to prison was pardoned by the President a day later. The editor of the government controlled paper, *The Chronicle*, who had revealed the story was promoted to a new post with no clearly defined duties indicating the Government's displeasure at his exposure of corruption and, at the same time, signalling to other media workers that exposing ministers' corrupt activities was not prudent. The President's interference with the course of justice appeared to condone the use of public office for personal gain and went some way in legitimising such behaviour by those in public office.

One of the major problems of patrimonialism in the civil service is that it distorts and paralyses the efficient operation of bureaucratic institutions designed to operate on rational-legal principles. For example, it becomes imprudent for a public official to discipline his or her junior officer who is related to a senior politician and this reduces their authority and effectiveness in the organisation. It also promotes more indiscipline among subordinates and frustration and apathy in those in charge of public institutions, and of course organisational performance suffers. Some of the effects of patrimonialism on public administration will become evident in Chapters 6 and 7.

Mandaza (1991) argues that while civil groups such as academics, student movements, churches, and human rights organisations are increasingly calling on the political and administrative elite to be more accountable for their public activities, their success in this respect will be limited. He contends that the political leadership relies on the vote of the peasants who loyally support government even in the face of all out opposition from the urban masses and elite groups. Mandaza (1991) cites, in support of this, the electoral victory of the ruling party in the 1990 elections against an opposition party widely supported by the urban workers and the petit bourgeoisie comprising the professionals, academic elite, church leaders, human rights movements, student groups and emerging indigenous business persons. The ruling party won again in 1995, in spite of serious allegations of grabbing of land intended for resettlement by ministers and senior government officers, none of whom were punished.

Drawing from this argument, it follows that efforts by various social groups to force public institutions to be more accountable and transparent in their operations have a limited chance of success because they are comprised of small elite groups which have no impact on the electoral process in the country and which the government can effectively ignore. This has serious implications for issues such as patients rights, and effective regulation of health workers because, in the Zimbabwean context, they would be championed by the small elite who know their rights. The poor majority are more concerned with access to health care than with the quality of that access, particularly after the introduction of the ESAP.

Organisation of the Book

Chapter 2 outlines how the data for this book was collected, discussing in detail the research methodology adopted, including the sampling methods, data collection methods and ethical dilemmas encountered. Chapter 3 provides essential information on the development of both the health care sector and the medical profession under colonialism and reveals the extent to which the nature of medical autonomy in Zimbabwe is still influenced by policies and decisions made in the colonial era. Chapter 4 examines the policies formulated by the post-colonial government and analyses their potential impact on medical autonomy. Chapter 5 discusses the nature of clinical autonomy exercised by doctors at the Parirenyatwa Group of Hospitals and comparisons are continually made with the situation in other countries. Chapter 6 presents the research findings on the nature of economic autonomy for government employed physicians and Chapter 7 examines the nature of professional regulation of medical education, licensing, and medical discipline. Finally, Chapter 8 summarises the major findings of the study and discusses its contributions to current theories of professions.

2 The Research Process

Introduction

The aim of this chapter is to discuss the research process through which data on the nature of medical autonomy for government-employed physicians as well as on the origins and development of Zimbabwe's health service system were obtained. More specifically, the chapter discusses: the types of data sought; the choice of data collection methods; the process of gaining access; the research context; the sampling of respondents; the data collection process, comprising unstructured interviews, observation and document analysis; data analysis; and some of the problems and ethical dilemmas encountered during the research.

Types of Information Sought

The research aimed to obtain data to portray the nature of clinical and economic autonomy exercised by doctors employed on a full-time basis at the Parirenyatwa Group of Hospitals. In order to determine the nature of clinical autonomy, the data had to reveal any limits to decision-making in clinical practice; the origin of the limits, i.e. whether economic, cultural, legal, political and their impact on decision-making around patient care. Information on the nature of economic autonomy exercised by government-employed doctors was obtained by examining: the conditions of service for the different grades of doctors; their bargaining power in negotiating their conditions of service with employers; the nature of private practice in the country; and the opportunities for individual doctors of joining the private sector, or otherwise earning money outside government employment.

In addition, data had to inform on the role of the medical profession as a collective in the regulation of medical education, licensing and discipline. More specifically, there was a need to explore the role of the medical profession in determining the size of the medical school intake, the nature of the medical school curriculum, and licensing. The research also had to establish the role of the medical profession within the Health Professions Council, which is the body responsible for regulating the

36

medical profession and other registrable health professions, and ascertain its effectiveness, alongside that of other institutions involved in the regulation of the medical profession. Finally, it was necessary to acquire information on the development of the health care system and the medical profession during and after the colonial era.

Data Collection Methods

Even though the questions addressed in the book have been studied fairly comprehensively in developed western countries and an established theoretical agenda has emerged, this research was entering a new terrain in both empirical and theoretical terms in studying a developing country. I decided to carry out a qualitative in-depth study which would allow for the emergence of rich data and a meaningful depiction of the situation. A large scale survey was not advisable in the absence of a well mapped-out literature on medical autonomy in the post-colonial context. Moreover, the highly sensitive nature of the research meant that it was not possible to obtain a random sample of respondents.

In order to collect the comprehensive data that were necessary to address the research problem in its breadth and depth, I took note of Burgess's (1982:165) assertion that, 'no one method can yield the truth about a situation'. In-depth unstructured interviews, document analysis and observation appeared to be the most appropriate data collection methods for my research. I heeded Schatzman and Strauss's (1973:7) suggestion that the researcher should regard 'any method of inquiry as a system of strategies and operations designed - at any time - for getting answers to certain questions about events which interest him [her]'. A critical consideration of my research problem indicated that it could not be adequately addressed using one method alone, not only because all methods have inherent deficiencies (see Denzin, 1989; Silverman, 1985), but also because particular methods were suitable for providing answers to specific aspects of the problem. Triangulation eliminates some of the weaknesses of individual data collection methods which can often limit the reliability and validity of findings (Philips, 1971). In addition, it 'is a plan of action that will raise sociologists above the personal biases that stem from single methodologies' (Denzin, 1989:236). The actual process of triangulation adopted in the current research is explained within the discussion of individual data collection methods.

In view of the exploratory nature of the research, the unstructured interview was adopted as the principal data collection method because it is more flexible and appropriate for research into areas in which the researcher is not fully aware of all the issues which might arise. Interviews have the added advantage of being able to provide both general and detailed information on specialized issues (Fielding, 1993). Accordingly, interview guides were prepared using concepts and definitions identified during the process of reviewing the literature. In view of the fact that most of the literature pertains to developed countries, most of the questions were open-ended. Such questions have an advantage where 'the issue is complex, where the relevant dimensions are not known and where the process is being explored' (Stacey, 1969:80). While interviews could furnish useful data on events that occurred after independence, the colonial situation required document analysis because most of those who might feasibly be able to provide information were not available, having either died or left the country. Similarly, statistical data such as the number of medical personnel employed in the Ministry of Health and at the Parirenyatwa Group of Hospitals, and the exact dates on which certain events occurred could only be reliably obtained from documents. Sometimes documents were the sole source of information, but they were also used extensively to validate data obtained either from observation or from interviews. As will be discussed in detail later, state official and, private official biographies as well as media documents, were used extensively in the research. In some instances, information acquired through interviews had to be verified through non-participant observation. For example, most doctors complained about the lack of, or breakdown of diagnostic and surgical equipment, something which I was able to validate by visiting the hospital X-ray and Pathology departments and observing for myself (as will be discussed in more detail later in the chapter).

Negotiating Access

While developing the research, I was aware that the process of negotiating access in the health sector was going to consist of what Johnson (1976:77) has described as a multistage 'progressive entree'. Any health related research carried out in Zimbabwe has to pass through the Medical Research Council (MRC) and the Ministry of Health and Child Welfare, in addition to negotiating access with the gatekeepers of the specific research setting where the field work takes place and obtaining the consent of individual respondents. This process has been known to take one full year and, not surprisingly, some researchers have abandoned their research due to frustration with the process. With this in mind, I initiated my negotiations to obtain permission six months before I was due to start fieldwork, in July of 1993.

However, a month later, I was informed by the Secretary to the Council that I had not been granted permission because my proposed research had policy implications and the Council does not approve such research unless it is for the benefit of government, my use of qualitative methodology was non-scientific, and the fact that even though I am a Zimbabwean, I was registered with a foreign university meant that I had to go through the Scientific Research Council before the MRC could consider my application. The Council's reaction was contrary to Abrams' observation that powerful gate-keepers prefer research that is relevant to the policy making process (Abrams, 1981 cited in Renzetti and Lee, 1993). Even under normal circumstances, carrying out research on powerful groups is difficult, as Spencer (1992) points out after his study of bureaucratic elites at West Point. Zimbabwean physicians are not easily accessible for research purposes at the best of times, but this was further complicated over the period during which I carried out my field work, since the medical profession was constantly in the media limelight over alleged malpractice involving a senior consultant anaesthetist whose case was already in the High Court. Clearly, my proposed research topic fell squarely into the category described by Lee and Renzetti (1993) as 'sensitive research'. The Medical Research Council, which includes physicians, was, I strongly suspect, protecting the interests of a powerful group by suppressing research which could reveal negative information detrimental to the group's interests.

I realised that my chances of securing access through the Medical Research Council were bleak. Fortunately, while I was still considering other possibilities, an option which I had not entertained, that of sponsorship by a powerful political patron, presented itself to me quite unexpectedly. Hoffman (1980) points out that access to influential elites can be obtained through the sponsorship of social acquaintances and personal contacts (cited in Hammersley and Atkinson, 1983). In my own research, I met by chance, the wife of a powerful government minister whom I had previously worked with, and explained my predicament and she offered to help. I subsequently submitted my application to her husband and permission was granted by the Ministry of Health and Child Welfare in less than a week. I was granted access to all health institutions, although I had to negotiate with individual respondents for permission to interview them. This experience was very similar to Cassell's who tried unsuccessfully for over a year to obtain permission to study surgeons in the United States and finally managed through the help of a friend who happened to be a chief surgeon (Cassell, 1988, cited in Hornsby-Smith, 1993).

Securing permission to enter my proposed research setting, the Parirenyatwa Group of Hospitals was easier as I had previously worked with the Medical Superintendent, the main gatekeeper, on an earlier research project and after showing him my letter from the Ministry of Health and explaining the nature of my research, I was granted access. I could enter the hospital wards and departments at any time, but was advised that interviews with individual physicians were best carried out outside the wards to minimise conflict with the heads of departments and disruption of operational routines in the hospital. The process of gaining access was clearly multistage involving negotiation with various gatekeepers of data sources and institutions and as described below, individual medical and non-medical respondents.

Research Setting

The choice of the research setting, a hospital, was largely determined by the nature of my research problem, which was to examine the nature of autonomy for different grades of government-employed doctors working in a clinical capacity. It had to be a government hospital employing a considerable number of physicians at different stages in their careers, that is: junior doctors; government medical officers; registrars; and consultants. Even though Harare Hospital, the only other central hospital in the capital city, has the same variety of doctors, it does not have a wide variety of patients, since it does not cater for private patients and their physicians. Thus, some of the major problems that have arisen in the mid-1990s between the government and medical doctors over the use of government beds for private patients, and allegations that government doctors spend more time with their own private patients admitted to the hospital, do not arise at Harare Hospital. Another important reason for selecting the Parirenyatwa Group of Hospitals was its convenience for me, both in terms of obtaining permission to carry out research and also in terms of geographical location from my residential base during field work.

Site Location

The Parirenyatwa Group of Hospitals is located on the northern side of the city of Harare, a distance of about two kilometres from the city centre. Unlike its sister, Harare Hospital, which is located adjacent to a big industrial area, Parirenyatwa is located in a high-income, low density, very expensive and now largely diplomatic residential area. It is easily accessible from the affluent northern residential suburbs for whose residents it was originally intended.

Historical Origins

The Old Central Hospital (formerly known as the Central Hospital), which is the oldest within the Parirenyatwa Group of Hospitals, was built on the present site in 1914 and gradually expanded as the settler population grew. The Annexe, (formerly known as The Lady Chancellor Maternity Hospital) was built on the same site in 1928 and converted into a nervous disorders hospital in 1957 after a new maternity hospital of the same name (now Mbuya Nehanda Maternity Hospital) was opened in 1955. Princess Margaret Hospital (now Sekuru Kaguvi Hospital, an eye unit) was built for the Asian and 'Coloured' population in 1955. The first phase of the new Andrew Fleming Hospital (now Parirenyatwa Hospital) was commissioned in 1974 and was built in five phases, the last of which was completed in 1982.

Before independence, three of the five hospitals in the then Salisbury Group of Hospitals (now Parirenyatwa Group of Hospitals) served the White community in and around the city of Salisbury (now Harare), while Harare Central Hospital was the ultimate referral centre for the Blacks, and Princess Margaret Hospital was for the 'Coloured' and Asian communities. Andrew Fleming Hospital was the ultimate referral centre for the White population in the country. Specialties such as cardiac surgery, renal dialysis and sophisticated radiotherapy were and are still only found in this hospital. Before independence, blacks who needed such treatment were admitted in the teaching wing of the Andrew Fleming Hospital (now Parirenyatwa Hospital) comprising 350 out of the 1,350 total beds in the hospital.

The 1,350-bed Parirenyatwa Hospital (formerly Andrew Fleming Hospital) is a large sprawling building, four storeys high, built with concrete and red brick and flat roofed. When the first phase of the hospital was commissioned in 1974, it was described as the largest and most sophisticated treatment centre in the country, comparing favourably with major hospitals

41

anywhere in the world. Over twenty years later, even though some of the linoleum wall covering and floor tiles are worn out, it remains quite impressive.

The completed hospital complex has all the medical specialties and other paramedical facilities that one expects in a big urban hospital and the only medical school in the country is also located in the hospital. In addition to providing facilities for undergraduate and post graduate medical teaching, the hospital complex also provides training facilities for technologists, occupational therapists, pharmacists, radiographers, basic nurse training, and post-basic nurse training in anaesthetics, theatre, intensive care, community nursing, nurse education and nursing administration. In the same location, but a few yards from the medical school, are the residential halls for medical students in their clinical training stage, and apartments for interns or house officers and other doctors entitled to hospital accommodation.

The Management Structure

The Salisbury Hospitals Act of 1975 established the Salisbury Hospital Board of Governors to administer the five hospitals which constituted the Salisbury Group of Hospitals (now Parirenyatwa Group of Hospitals). The group comprised Princess Margaret Hospital (now Sekuru Kaguvi); Lady Chancellor Maternity Hospital (now Mbuya NeHanda); Andrew Fleming Hospital (now Parirenyatwa hospital); Annexe (now a psychiatric wing of the Parirenyatwa Group of Hospitals); the old central hospital (now a geriatric hospital); and Harare Central Hospital, the central hospital for Blacks located about ten kilometres away. The hospitals were managed and controlled by a Board comprising nineteen members appointed by and answerable to the Minister of Health from the following institutions: four suggested by the University of Rhodesia (now University of Zimbabwe) Council; three by the Rhodesia Medical Association (now ZMA); three by the medical school; and two by the Ministry of Health. The Minister appointed five non-medical members to the Board and the Medical Superintendent, a doctor by profession, was an *ex-officio* member of the Board. In addition, the Minister appointed an honorary consultant on the Board. Up to 1980, there were no less than eight physicians out of a total of nineteen board members. No other health occupations were represented on the Board, even though they, rather than physicians, were the full-time employees of the hospital. The 1975 Salisbury Hospitals Act defined the functions of the Board as to 'manage, and control the Salisbury Group of

Hospitals and to provide for its functions relating to the care and the treatment of the sick, medical education, and research' (Salisbury Hospitals Act, 1975:4). It had powers 'to provide for the transfer of certain moveable assets and certain liabilities...; to regulate the financial affairs thereof; to provide for the staffing of such hospitals; and to provide for matters incidental or connected with the foregoing' (Salisbury Hospitals Act, 1975:4).

According to the terms of the Medical Services Act (1979), the Board assumed the responsibility of determining the right of individual private practitioners to admit their patients to Andrew Fleming Hospital, the appointment of those who could work as consultants in the hospital, and the terms under which they worked in the hospital. In order to fulfil the above function and the regulation of financial affairs, the Board established medical appointments and finance committees respectively. The dominance of the medical profession in the hospital was further strengthened by the Act which stipulated that whenever the Board met, at least half of the members had to be doctors. The Act also opened Andrew Fleming hospital to non-white doctors granted access by the Salisbury Group of Hospitals Board.

In 1981, the first Minister of Health reduced the number of members appointed to the board by the University of Zimbabwe and the ZMA and, for the first time, nurses were represented. The board continued to function rather ineffectively until November 1992 when it was dissolved by the current Minister of Health who objected to the Board's decision to build a rudimentary hospital visitors' shelter where visitors could seek protection from the sun and rain while waiting for the hospital visiting hour. The Minister felt that the money could have been better used to procure hospital equipment. There were accusations and counter-accusations between the Minister of Health and the then Medical Superintendent of the Parirenyatwa Group of Hospitals, with the latter supported by the Board. This culminated in the resignation of the Chairperson of the Board, followed soon after by the Medical Superintendent in 1992 and after this, the rest of the Board ceased to function. The Minister of Health informed me in a personal interview that some of the Board members resigned, while others left when their term of office expired in November 1993. He appointed a technical committee comprising officials from the Ministry of Health and Parirenyatwa Hospital to perform the functions of the Board until a new board could be appointed. In personal interviews, some of the ex-Board members insisted that they were never formally informed about the status of the Board. As of August 1995, a new board had still not been appointed, even though the technical committee could not perform many of the functions of the Board because it did not have the legal mandate to do so. This gave the Minister near total control because all those appointed to the technical committee are Ministry of Health employees under his jurisdiction.

Sampling of Medical Doctors

The need for sampling of respondents has been raised by a number of social scientists who make the obvious point that one cannot interview everyone during the process of field work (Burgess, 1982). The categories of people for interview was determined by the research question, which sought to establish the nature of autonomy exercised by various grades of government-employed doctors working at Parirenyatwa Hospital. It was important to conduct interviews with a sample of junior doctors, comprising junior resident medical officers (JRMOs), senior resident medical officers (SRMOs) and senior house officers (SHOs); Government Medical Officers (GMOs); registrars; and consultants (see Figure 2.1 for the different grades of doctors at the hospital). My sampling frame therefore comprised all physicians employed on a full-time basis at Parirenyatwa Hospital, which turned out to be sixty (see Table 2.1). A much larger number of doctors attend patients at Parirenyatwa, but some are full-time private doctors tending their private patients, while others occupy shared posts with Harare Hospital. A large number of university-employed medical lecturers look after both their own and government patients, but they are not government employees. However, some were interviewed in their capacity as key informants, providing information on, for example, medical education and the Health Professions Council.

I decided to use convenience and snowball sampling to select medical respondents, but adopted purposive sampling and snowball sampling for the key informants. In the case of medical respondents, I was aware, from previous experience (MOH, 1991), that physicians are usually reluctant to be interviewed. In 1991, I carried out a study for the Ministry of Health to identify the causes of high turnover among professional health personnel and government-employed physicians were the most elusive group, partly because of time constraints, but also because they claimed to be afraid of victimization by government if they expressed a negative attitude about its health policies in interviews. The reaction, then, was understandable, in view of their experiences after the 1989 doctors' strike, which will be

Figure 2.1   Different Grades of Doctors Classified by Training and Experience

```
┌─────────────────────────────────────────────────────────────┐
│                          Consultant                          │
│   3 to 5 year specialist training at Masters degree level or │
│  membership of the Royal College in the United Kingdom and   │
│            experience working as Senior Registrar            │
└─────────────────────────────────────────────────────────────┘
                              │
┌─────────────────────────────────────────────────────────────┐
│                  Senior Registrar/Registrar                  │
│  Over 4 years post-graduate experience, and either passed Part I │
│    of membership of one of the Royal Colleges or nearing     │
│  completion of a Masters degree in one of the specialties in │
│                           Zimbabwe                           │
└─────────────────────────────────────────────────────────────┘
                              │
┌─────────────────────────────────────────────────────────────┐
│                 Junior Registrar/GMO/HMO                     │
│   Minimum of 3 years post-basic qualification experience     │
└─────────────────────────────────────────────────────────────┘
                              │
┌─────────────────────────────────────────────────────────────┐
│                 Senior House Officer (SHO)                   │
│                First year of work after internship           │
└─────────────────────────────────────────────────────────────┘
                              │
┌─────────────────────────────────────────────────────────────┐
│           Senior Resident Medical Officer (SRMO)             │
│                    Second year of internship                 │
└─────────────────────────────────────────────────────────────┘
                              │
┌─────────────────────────────────────────────────────────────┐
│           Junior Resident Medical Officer (JRMO)            │
│   First year of internship, following 5 years post-A Level   │
│                   university medical training               │
└─────────────────────────────────────────────────────────────┘
```

Table 2.1   Staff Establishment for the Parirenyatwa Group of Hospitals

Category	Required Number	Authorized Establishment	In Post	Vacant Posts
Physician	8-16	3	2	1
Paediatrician	10-20	2	0	2
Surgeon	12-24	4	4	0
Obstetrics + Gynaecology	4-8	3	0	3
Anaesthetist	8-16	6	2	4
Opthmology	4-8	3	1	2
Radiology	3-6	3	1	2
Radiotherapy	4-8	0	2	-
Pathology	6-12	3	3	0
Rehabilitation Medicine	2-4	0	1	0
Public Health	2-4	0	0	0
Registrar	50-100	27	15	12
JRMO/SRMO	50-100	53	12	42
HMO	8-16	5	6	0
GMO	10-20	9	11	0
Nurse	820-1640	701	692	9
Dental Surgeon	2-4	0	0	0
Pharmacist	8-16	10	8	2
Radiographer	40-80	40	26	14
Laboratory Technician	60-120	100	99	1
Physiotherapist	20-40	18	7	11
Occupational Therapist	10-20	1	0	1
Speech Therapy	3-6	0	0	0
Equipment Technician	20-40	6	6	0

Source: Report on Policy and Management of Parirenyatwa Group of Hospitals, MOH & CW Technical Committee, 1994, pp. 35-36.

described in Chapter 6. In addition, they complained that many studies carried out on them did not seem to benefit them as a group in any way and, not surprisingly, there was a very poor response to both face-to-face interviews and postal questionnaires in the 1991 study.

In view of this, I opted for convenience and snowball sampling. I surmised that respondents selected this way could be just as representative as those selected using random sampling methods, assuming that the groups of SRMOs, JRMOs and SHOs were fairly homogenous groups who were likely to share many views and experiences. The basis of this assumption was that, firstly; they trained as a cohort during the seven years of medical education, and for the last five of those years they were isolated from non-medical university students. Their lecture rooms and their residential accommodation are located in the grounds of the Parirenyatwa Hospital complex, six kilometres from the main campus where non-medical students have their lecture rooms and residential accommodation. My assumption that a non-random sample with shared values is as representative as a random sample is endorsed by Honigmann (1982:89) who argues that 'the more homogenous the universe, the more likely it is that probability and non-probability samples will manifest similar characteristics and results'. Further still, Mead (1953) maintains that non-random sampling methods are logical as long as one is not trying to answer 'how often' and 'how much', but wants to address qualitative problems. But, as pointed out above, the main reason for adopting non-random samples was their suitability in the Zimbabwean context.

If all junior doctors more-or-less shared the same values, I could interview those who were agreeable or had the time whenever I approached them. The assumption of shared values did not extend to registrars and consultants, most of whom either obtained their first degrees or post-graduate degrees abroad and with equally varied work experiences. In their case, convenience sampling was adopted because they were even more reluctant than the junior doctors to make appointments for interviews. Unlike junior doctors who live in the hospital grounds, senior doctors live in their private accommodation all over the residential suburbs. As the universe from which I was to draw the sample of medical respondents only comprised sixty doctors, I aimed to interview at least 50 percent of every grade of doctors in the hospital.

For the selection of JRMOs, SRMOs and SHOs, I approached the President and Secretary-General of the Hospital Doctors Association (HDA) to inform them of the research and enlist their support. They became unofficial gatekeepers, asking me for letters of clearance from the Medical Research Council, the Ministry of Health and the Parirenyatwa Group of Hospitals' Medical Superintendent. Having their support turned out to be quite useful, as junior doctors became more cooperative and helpful whenever I informed them that I had the blessing of both the President and the Secretary-General of their association. I was in fact, able to interview all the junior doctors based at Parirenyatwa, including both the President and Secretary-General of the HDA who were better informed on some issues than other junior doctors due to their role as spokespersons of the junior doctors.

In drawing samples of hospital medical officers (HMO), and general medical officers (GMO) and registrars, I obtained names from the duty rosters in the wards, and then phoned the wards, waited for them outside theatre and in the out-patients department after clinics in order to secure interviews. They were the most difficult grades to secure interviews with because they are quite busy in the hospital, especially as consultants leave much of their workload to them. Most of them also practise privately. Unlike consultants who have offices in the hospital and listed phone numbers of their private surgeries, once GMOs, HMOs and registrars leave the hospital, they are very difficult to locate. Out of the thirty two HMOs, GMOs and registrars based at Parirenyatwa Hospital, I was able to secure ten interviews out of the eighteen requests that I made.

As I had initially feared, scheduling interviews with consultants was very difficult primarily because, in addition to their workload in the government hospital, they also have surgeries where they see their private patients. Attempts were made to schedule interviews either through their secretaries in the government hospital or at their private surgeries. Two of the consultants were out of the country and another four were expatriates and only four of the ten consultants that I approached were prepared to fix firm appointments. Most explained that they could not possibly see me for more than fifteen minutes because they were far too busy but fortunately, when I did hold the interviews with the four, each of them exceeded an hour. In addition, I had one group interview with three consultants whom I approached in the University senior common room one evening, and I was able to fix an additional individual interview with one of them who was also a ZMA representative. So, in total I was able to carry out five individual interviews and one group interview comprising three consultants at Parirenyatwa Hospital.

Sampling of Key Informants and Non-medical Respondents

In the selection of key informants, the most appropriate methods were purposive and snowball sampling because informants were selected for the special information which they had by virtue of the positions they occupied in the health care system. Some of the essential information I required to address the research problem fully could only be obtained in interviews with current and previous holders of specific positions in either the Ministry of Health or other health-related organizations. The selection of key informants and other non-medical officials was determined by the nature of the organizations which they worked for. While reviewing literature and reading about the medical profession and the health services in Zimbabwe, I identified the relevant organizations and decided to interview one or two of the most senior persons in each organisation, depending on the information that they were able to provide.

In some instances, the person selected was not necessarily the most senior, but was strategically located and was able to provide what Tremblay (1982) has called 'broad general information', while others were chosen for their roles and perspectives (Strauss, 1964), and still others were selected for the fine detail and specialized information which they could provide, as suggested by Spradley (1979) and Tremblay (1982).

The organizations that were identified include: the Ministry of Health; the Health Professions Council; the Consumer Council of Zimbabwe; the Zimbabwe Medical Association; the Hospital Doctors' Association; the College of Primary Care Physicians; the University of Zimbabwe Medical School; the Zimbabwe Nurses' Association; the Zimbabwe National Association of Traditional Healers (ZINATHA); and ZimRights (local human rights organisation). The offices of these organizations were visited and the relevant officials were identified. There was no pre-determination of the number of individuals interviewed in any one organisation, as this depended on the comprehensiveness of the information provided by the first interviewee. Some respondents were suggested to me by others who often pointed out that someone else was better informed about issues that I raised. Thus, key informants were able to provide valuable insights into certain issues, and, at the same time, suggest what Yin (1994 :84) has referred to as 'corroboratory evidence' and, in some cases, provide access to such sources. Most questions were posed to several people in similar and different professional and organisational positions.

Some of the key informants had multiple roles, or they previously held positions in other organizations and were therefore able to provide extensive and detailed information on many issues central to the research. For example, the current Minister of Health, Dr Timothy Stamps, is a former president of the College of Primary Care Physicians. Similarly, the current president of the Health Professions Council is a senior surgeon, one of the longest serving black medical lecturers, a member of the medical curriculum review committee, and a former dean of the Faculty of Medicine. I was also able to interview two former Permanent Secretaries for Health, both of whom covered a wide range of key areas pertaining to both the colonial and post-colonial era.

Altogether, I interviewed sixty-six respondents, including medical doctors and key informants and held three group discussions. The group discussions were not planned, but during the Kadoma Workshop, which will be discussed later in the chapter, I had the opportunity to discuss the nature of medical practice in Zimbabwe on two separate occasions. One group comprised five people: a medical superintendent of a provincial hospital, a matron of a central hospital, the national Director of Nursing Services, a medical lecturer and two nurses from a provincial hospital. The other group comprised a representative of the Zimbabwe Nurses' Association (ZINA), the Director of Maternal and Child Health in the Ministry of Health (a medical doctor by training), one officer from the Planning and Training Section of the Ministry of Health, and the President of the Zimbabwe Association of Church-related Hospitals (ZACH). The third group comprising three consultants has already been described.

Unstructured Interviews

Some aspects of the research process described took place simultaneously. For example, while I was trying to secure access, I was also in the process of collecting documentary evidence and interviewing a number of key informants. Importantly, at this time junior doctors went on strike (described in detail in Chapter 6) before I had interviewed any of them, and I decided to carry out the interviews on the assumption that they would now have more time on their hands. When I approached the hospital to make contact with the doctors, over sixty junior doctors from both Harare and Parirenyatwa hospitals were standing in the grounds of the doctors' residences where they spent most of their mornings waiting for news on the government's reaction to the strike and later for news on the progress of the negotiations between government and the HDA executive.

I decided to approach a group of three women doctors standing at the edge of the gathering and introduced myself in a friendly but subdued manner. Approaching men first could have portrayed me as 'too forward' to both male and female groups and could have aroused both suspicion and hostility. I explained the nature of my research, informed them that the HDA was supportive and then asked whether they would be willing to be interviewed. Initially they were quite sceptical but I reassured them that I was not from the Ministry of Health and because some of their own lecturers were opposed to the strike, I also down-played my connection with the University of Zimbabwe, stressing instead that I was studying at a foreign University. I assured them that the information that they provided would be confidential and, as a last resort, showed them my Warwick University identity card and further pointed out that they need not introduce themselves to me by name if they did not feel comfortable with that. Two of the doctors agreed, but the third one explained that talking about the strike would raise her 'blood pressure'.

I was able to interview one of the respondents there and then, but scheduled an interview for a few days later with the second one. After that first interview, my informant and I approached the biggest group of male doctors and again renegotiated access, stating the objective of my study as 'finding out why doctors are leaving government hospitals'. I quickly found that both doctors and other informants were more receptive to a research topic that was relevant to their existing problems. Most of those I approached expressed a willingness to be interviewed, but many explained that they had locum jobs lined up, and that I should make appointments to interview them later. In fact most of them did locum work during this period to the extent that even their negotiating teams changed members almost on a daily basis because everyone wanted to take advantage of this time to make some money and only the President of HDA attended all of the negotiation meetings.

I got into the habit of going to the hospital doctors' residence every morning and approaching a group with someone that I had interviewed before. Even though the HDA executive held meetings with striking doctors almost daily to brief them on developments, I was not allowed access to those meetings. I was able to carry out interviews with five JRMOs and SRMOs and two HSOs during the strike period and arranged for a further five which took place later.

One of the most important issues which I had to address during the course of my field work was the anonymity and confidentiality of my respondents and the information that they provided. Junior doctors, in particular, were concerned that their identities should not be revealed in case they were victimized. The strike made the research topic even more sensitive due to what Lee (1993) has referred to as situational and socio-political reasons. Junior doctors were worried about the possibility of a backlash by the government, which was understandable and not totally unexpected given that during the last doctors' strike in 1989, some of the strikers had been arrested. They agreed to be interviewed, but categorically stated that tape-recording of the interviews was unacceptable, and I had no option but to respect their wishes. The interviews were already what Lee (1993) has described as an 'intrusive threat' and the least I could do in the face of their own generosity in granting me interviews was not to push or resort to the unethical use of a hidden tape-recorder. To reassure them of anonymity of the information obtained, I reiterated that they did not have to reveal their names to me if they did not want to, and in fact, most did not introduce themselves by name, which indicated that they were genuinely worried about the possibility of victimization if the information and their identity were revealed.

Fortunately, all the informants agreed to note-taking while interviews were in progress. Even the Minister of Health mentioned several times that some aspects of his interview were strictly off the record. The wariness that Zimbabwean people have about tape-recording interviews was brought home to me by one key informant, a surgeon and lecturer in the medical school and my very last informant. By the time his interview was conducted, I had totally given up on the idea of tape-recording because everyone so far had refused. When I took out my note book and asked whether he would mind if I took notes he asked, 'Why are you, a sociologist, not recording this interview?' I explained that everyone else had refused and I had since abandoned the idea. He assured me that he was not worried about tape recording and had long ceased caring about the activities of the Central Intelligence Organisation because he was sure that they already had a fat dossier on him. Whenever he said something critical of the government, he would jokingly repeat, 'Did you get that?' to an imaginary tape recorder supposedly hidden by the much feared and much maligned intelligence service. This indicated to me that in spite of his nonchalant attitude about the possibility of the information getting into the 'wrong hands', the thought was never far from his mind. Much of the information would not be considered sensitive in other contexts, but in Zimbabwe, it was sensitive, reinforcing Lee's (1993) point that sensitivity is contextual.

All of the interview data were recorded by long and short hand and later transcribed. An attempt was made to record everything that was said and, fortunately, the respondents did not mind that I was writing, and in fact, quite often would stop talking when I appeared not to be writing something down. My note-taking skills improved progressively so that most of the interview proceedings were recorded almost verbatim. Note-taking obviously cannot be as efficient as tape-recording, in which pauses and sighs and other verbal cues are recorded. The one disadvantage was that in some instances, I failed to follow up a question immediately which I would probably have done had I not been paying so much attention to recording, but luckily, this did not occur often and, in some cases, I had repeat interviews with the same respondents to clarify issues raised in the first interview and to discuss other issues of interest. In most cases, any interesting or unexpected issues that arose were raised in subsequent interviews with other respondents and, as a result, interviews got more comprehensive as the field work progressed.

In the course of the interviews, an attempt was made to ensure that information obtained could answer the questions posed, but respondents were allowed to dwell on issues as they chose, and consequently, the sequence varied across interviews. I followed Burgess's (1982:107) advice to 'probe deeply, to uncover new clues, to open up new dimensions of a problem and to secure vivid, accurate inclusive accounts'. Consequently, the length of my interviews varied, ranging from thirty minutes to three hours, with most over an hour in length, but interviews with some of the key informants took several sessions because of time constraints, with repeat interviews adding up to six hours with one respondent. The interviews in these and other similar cases were extensive and detailed, covering many key areas commensurate with an informant's roles.

I held numerous informal discussions with many people in the Ministry of Health and many other organizations which were visited in the course of carrying out the research. Fortunately, most people in Zimbabwe are so informal that passengers in buses, and other public places generally debate whatever issue is topical in the media at that point in time. I listened avidly to these debates with the intention of gauging the public's response, particularly to the doctors' strike, the state of the health services, the newly introduced hospital fees and the McGowan malpractice case. I recorded the information obtained in this way when I was on my own and it provided me with a comprehensive perspective of the issues under investigation. I became quite adept at seizing any opportunities for gathering data for my research and one such occasion is described below.

Kadoma Workshop

I had the rare opportunity of attending a workshop organised by the Ministry of Health to draft a Patients' Rights Charter, in a small town called Kadoma, two hundred kilometres outside Harare. My attendance occurred fortuitously, as the workshop was only meant for senior officials and representatives of all health-related organizations comprising: the Ministry of Health; the private medical sector; the city health departments; the mission hospitals; the health insurance organisations; the Zimbabwe Nurses' Association; the Consumer Council of Zimbabwe; ZimRights; the Zimbabwe Medical Association; the College of Primary Care Physicians, representatives of the pharmaceutical industry; and doctors and nurses from the various provinces. I happened to be in the Ministry of Health trying to arrange an appointment with one of the officials, when I overheard his secretary making telephone calls to the workshop participants and informing them of travel arrangements. I convinced the organisers of the need to have a paper discussing patients' views of the government health services which I could deliver. I was invited on the condition that I did not publicize the conditions under which I was attending.

The workshop was extremely useful for me because most participants presented papers on how their organizations would contribute to the planned Patients' Rights Charter. Specifically, the Ministry of Health explained what they expected to achieve with the charter and why it had been found necessary to have one. In addition, the Ministry unveiled its proposed health insurance scheme and provided the rationale for the introduction of hospital fees. Participants took the opportunity to discuss problems in the Ministry of Health, which candidly accepted some responsibility, but also defended itself vigorously and there was no evasion of questions by the officials, who appeared to be genuinely interested in making health institutions more responsive and user-friendly.

This workshop provided me with an opportunity to talk directly to policy-makers and heads of institutions and government departments without too much formality and having to negotiate and renegotiate with various gatekeepers for access. I had my first extensive interview with the president of ZMA during the workshop, without which I would have had to travel six hundred kilometres to interview him in Bulawayo (see Figure 1.1). I received official documents like other participants and when I explained my area of research, some participants referred me to potential sources of information, in the form of other respondents and documentary sources. I held impromptu discussions in pairs or in groups during tea, lunch and dinner breaks, ensuring that I met different people or groups each time. These discussions greatly enriched and gave depth to my understanding of the health care sector and medical practice in Zimbabwe. I was careful to pay equal attention to male and female participants, as advised by Easterday *et al* (1982), which was not always to my advantage because most policy makers and heads of institutions are male. I also took Easterday *et al's* (1982) advice to maintain a cordial but distant relationship with male respondents so that there was no misunderstanding and 'hustling'.

The April/May 1994 Doctors' Strike

The outbreak of the doctors' strike during the course of my field work was another serendipitous, but critical development which generated a wealth of crucial data and greatly facilitated the analysis of the relationship between the state and the medical profession. The doctors went on strike on the 15th of April 1994 to back a demand for better salaries and allowances, the details will be discussed in Chapter 6. The strike provided a rare opportunity for me to witness the two sides, i.e. the government and the hospital-based medical doctors, in open conflict. I was able to observe events first hand, interview the participants, analyze newspaper reports and journals at the time of their production, judge the accuracy of media reports and assess the mood of the public and the opinion-makers. The strike afforded me an opportunity to examine: the channels of communication between the Ministry of Health and the HDA; the decision-making processes in government; the negotiation process; the feelings and behaviour of the doctors; the inter- and intra-professional relations among the different grades of government doctors and other sectors of the medical profession working in the city council, university, private sector and other health workers. I was also able to assess the impact of the strike on hospital services at Parirenyatwa. This 'untoward event' had a far reaching impact on subsequent research effort and the conclusions drawn.

Observation

Non-participant observation was also used as a mode of data collection in the research, being particularly useful for validating data obtained through interviews (as suggested by Bell, 1993). One of the aims of the observation was verification of complaints made by doctors of all grades about the breakdown and shortage of some essential equipment such as X-ray machines, laboratory equipment, linen and gloves. I was also able to confirm the complaints about the long queues which doctors had to contend with, particularly in the Eye Unit.

This research is not about patients, the organisation of work in the hospital or even the work patterns of individual doctors, but is concerned with assessing the extent to which doctors are able to make autonomous decisions in their work, which is not something which I could ascertain by observation. Observation was not the principal data collection method, but as mentioned above, it was useful in acquainting me with the setting in which doctors work, giving me the 'feel of the place', and validating data obtained from other sources. As a trained nurse, I was able to use my own experience to assess some of the conditions in the hospital. For example, when doctors talked of a shortage of nurses, I was able to confirm this after looking at the duty rosters of some of the wards.

In order to discover the state of the equipment in the X-ray department, I visited it twice during the course of my field work, once in February and once during the doctors' strike in April, which radiographers joined in sympathy. I was able to confirm for myself that more than 50 percent of the machines were not working and that the department was short-staffed, with only twenty-six of the forty radiographer posts occupied. I observed the long queues of patients waiting to be attended to and I also chatted to three of the radiographers. I also visited the Pathology Department twice, once in April 1994 to interview the senior registrar and once during the doctors' strike, which laboratory technologists and technicians joined in support of the doctors. On the first occasion, the registrar took me round to show me the state of the equipment in the laboratories and explain why technicians were not able to work as efficiently and as speedily as was expected of them. I visited the Central Sterilizing Department (CSSD) responsible for sterilizing all the equipment, linen and gloves in the hospital in March to check out the sterilizing equipment, which had allegedly been out of order for a number of years.

I was able to observe the Casualty and Outpatients departments more often because both are on the entrance to the main hospital. I sat among the patients in Casualty for two hours on two occasions to see how long patients actually wait before they are attended to and once during the doctors' strike. I visited the Eye Clinic twice in the morning in May in order to assess the workload about which the doctors had complained and also to check its medical staff establishment.

Two surgical, two paediatric and one gynaecological wards were visited in March 1994 but, I was not able to stay long and observe because the wards were busy and the sisters reluctantly agreed to have me there outside visiting hours. It was during these periods that I observed the state of ward equipment and supplies of linen. Data obtained through observation were extremely important in validating information that was obtained in interviews and from documentary sources, such as the report of the Ministry of Health Technical Committee at Parirenyatwa and reports of the parliamentary committees investigating the state of the government health institutions. These documents describe the state of Parirenyatwa Hospital in 1992/3 and 1994 and through observation, I was able to assess the extent to which things had improved, deteriorated or remained constant.

Documentary Sources

Documents were one of the principal sources of data in this research. They were valuable as sources of historical information and for purposes of triangulation, as advocated by Denzin (1989) and Schatzman and Strauss (1973). They were used as sources of information which could not be 'reached' in any other way (Hakim, 1987; Lofland and Lofland, 1984:12), such as events that occurred in the early history of the country, but they were also useful as a source of reference on contemporary events. For example, it was one of the government-controlled newspapers which revealed that HDA negotiators changed with every meeting, but the reason for this was assumed to be fear of victimization for the few members of the executive. It was only after I raised this with two members of the HDA executive in interviews that I was informed of the real reason, earning money in locum work.

As part of my field work, I collected state official documents, private official documents, mass media publications, and personal biographies. Documents were obtained from various organizations which include: the Ministry of Health; the Government Publishers; the University of Zimbabwe Medical School; the National Archives; the Parliament; the Zimbabwe Congress of Trade Unions; the Zimbabwe Medical Association; the Zimbabwe Nurses' Association; the Hospital Doctors' Association; Zimbabwe News Agency; the Ministry of Information; and the Zimbabwe International Association of News Agents. Documents, like other sources of research data, have their strengths and weaknesses and for this reason, each documentary source was evaluated in terms of authenticity, credibility, representativeness, and meaning (Scott, 1990). Authenticity refers to how genuine the documents are, in terms of being valid copies of the original and being clear of accidental or deliberate adulteration in the process of reproduction.

Scott (1990) expresses the need to establish whether documents studied are representative or typical of those available in order to determine the extent to which reliable conclusions can be drawn from them, something which may be difficult to achieve because of problems of access and availability (Scott, 1990). In my case, for example, I was not able to establish the representativeness of some documents, as will be explained below, because there was no inventory indicating how many documents relevant to my research were available in most of the different organizations which held them. I did not sample those which I had access to, but rather examined all that appeared relevant to my research.

Finally, Scott (1990) emphasizes the need to establish that the researcher understands the cultural and contextual meanings of events from documents. Documentary sources are 'socially situated products' and the meaning intended by the author can be different from the meaning imputed to it by the reader, with the gap between the two widening with increased social differentiation of the author and the researcher or reader (Scott, 1990: 34). Scott's point struck me when reading some of the biographical books written by Gelfand, the most distinguished medical doctor in Zimbabwe and the founder and editor of the *Central African Medical Journal* until his death in 1985. His interpretation of some events that he describes differs from my own, which I attribute to differences in our social backgrounds, and other socio-demographic factors. Gelfand was a white missionary, a professor of medicine, a champion of private medical practice, and an important member of the colonial society. His praise for some men who were die-hard racists and his own silence on the issue of colonialism and the inequalities in the society of which he was a member, make it difficult for me to agree with his portrayal of some people and events. I am a black woman who grew up and reached adulthood under racial oppression and inequality.

One very noticeable factor is that the historical accounts on the development of the health services reflect a masculine construction of social reality. The Rhodesian and Zimbabwean health care sector which they portray was established and maintained by men, even though the largest group of health workers were and still are female nurses. There is very little mention of women, except for the odd obituaries of female doctors and pictures of graduating nurses, or some other such marginal occasion. This is not only a reflection of the gender of the authors and the patriarchal nature of the society, but also of the fact that men occupied and continue to hold the top administrative posts in the health care system, as in every other sector of Rhodesian/Zimbabwean society (Gelfand did acknowledge the role of women in mission health institutions in his last book, *Godly Medicine in Zimbabwe*, 1988).

State Official Documents

The state official documents analyzed include: the Hansard; various health acts; national economic plans; Ministry of Health annual plans and other administrative documents; parliamentary and ministerial investigative reports; ministerial speeches; and proceedings of government health-related workshops. In some instances, the existence of a document was mentioned during an interview and sometimes documents were referred to in other documents. My assessment of the state official documents is that they were all authentic copies of the original ones. In most instances, I obtained the original document and copied it myself, while others were copied for me by the staff at the National Archives, as is standard practice.

I was refused access to documents pertaining to patient complaints and those outlining medical disciplinary cases that have come before the Health Professions Council, and so had to rely heavily on information from interviews and secondary sources, such as the Report of the Parliamentary Select Committee on the HPC and newspaper articles. The disadvantage, as with other secondary sources, is that their focus was different from mine and I had to extrapolate what was relevant for me. To compensate for this, I was able to interview the secretary to the Committee extensively and he was able to provide me with some of the information which was missing from the report. Documents were only one of several other data collection methods, so their weaknesses were certainly minimized, if not nullified, by information obtained through other methods.

Analyses of colonial and post-colonial official government documents clearly indicate the different orientations of the two eras and were very useful for the historical chapter of the thesis. I studied in detail the health acts; debates on the annual budget; the financial estimates for the Ministry of Health; reports of Parliamentary investigation of the Service Ministries Committee on the Ministry of Health; and parliamentary and ministerial commissioned reports.

Private Official Documents

Private official documents refer to documents that belong to private but formal organizations (Scott, 1990), such as professional associations like HDA and ZMA. The documents embraced policy statements, constitutions and proceedings of meetings and workshops of these organizations. The *Central African Medical Journal (CAJM)* is a privately owned but formal journal which was founded and edited by Professor Gelfand and his wife for thirty years and is now run by charitable trust. I also examined periodic newsletters produced by the University of Rhodesia/Zimbabwe Medical Students' Association for information on the health care system and medical practice during and after the colonial era. Fortunately, the *Central African Medical Journal* always published summaries of minutes of meetings of the local branch of the British Medical Association (later the Rhodesia Medical Association) and the Medical Dental and Allied Professions Council and parliamentary proceedings relating to medical practice in the country. The editions produced during the colonial era were very useful on depicting the relationship between the state and the medical profession. Unfortunately, after the death of Professor Gelfand in 1985, the journal stopped publishing minutes of ZMA, HPC and parliamentary proceedings.

I had access to the minutes of meetings of the Hospital Doctors' Association, starting from its inception in 1986 until 1994. These files proved quite useful as they contained all the minutes of the meetings ever held, as well as copies of correspondence between the executive committee of HDA and the Ministry of Health, the Zimbabwe Medical Association, Zimbabwe Nurses' Association, the College of Primary Care Physicians and its members. The HDA files provided very comprehensive information which enabled me to reconstruct the 1988, 1989 and 1994 strikes. I did not have access to the minutes of the Zimbabwe Medical Association meetings from 1985 onwards, but obtained a number of policy documents. Similarly, I received limited documents from the College of Primary Care Physicians and the Zimbabwe Nurses' Association, but had comprehensive interviews with the presidents of all the organizations.

Public Media Publications

I searched all the national daily and weekly newspapers, and weekly and monthly magazines published after independence for information relevant to my research. Newspapers were very helpful in portraying the changeover in the government itself. Even though the main newspapers which had supported the colonial government were bought by the government after independence, in the first few years a number of the reporters from the colonial era were still in office and their critical attitude to the new health policies is quite evident. Over the years this has been replaced by sycophantic articles which tend to dwell on the activities of the government officials and are generally less critical.

Independent newspapers, such as the *Financial Gazette*, which was a bit muted in its criticism of government in the first few years of independence, has now become very critical and relishes revealing information embarrassing to the government or its officers. The *Financial Gazette* and a few other monthly magazines such as *Horizon* and *Moto* analyze and reveal the behaviour of politicians, as well as government policies, including the woes of the health sector. Some of them have been used as a mouth piece by the medical profession on a number of issues. Letters to the editors were a good barometer of the public's response to government policies, reaction to the strikes and of the general mood and perceptions of the different social groups in Zimbabwe. The obvious biases of the newspapers arising from their ownership meant that I had to validate any information that I obtained with data from other sources.

Personal Biographies

In addition to the other documentary sources, biographies, which include *Tropical Victory* (Gelfand, 1953), *Huggins of Rhodesia* (Gann and Gelfand, 1964), *The Fleming Letters* (Gelfand, 1959); *A Service to the Sick* (Gelfand, 1976); and *Godly Medicine in Zimbabwe* (Gelfand, 1988) were extremely useful in providing historical information from individual personal accounts of the early doctors and settlers. Although they are all authentic and credible sources of information, it was difficult to establish how representative they are. For example all of the above, except the last one, were published outside the country and are not available in public libraries in Zimbabwe, and there may be many other similarly inaccessible publications. Gelfand was a committed physician and did a lot to enhance the image of the profession, but he was also quite uncritical of it. In the thirty years that he was editor of the *CAJM*, he did not once criticize the medical profession and even when one physician was guilty of gross malpractice for which other doctors thought he would be imprisoned, there was no editorial comment. Even Gelfand's books on missionary medicine depict most missionaries as living saints, while other sources, such as Van Onselen (1976) show that a number of church leaders were less than holy, to say the least. The reason for not reporting negative cases was probably to ensure that the medical profession retained a good reputation abroad. This confirms Plummer's argument that 'most writings ... are context-bound and speak to certain people, times and circumstances' (Plummer, 1983:14). *A Central African Odyssey* (Cowen, 1995), a book on medical practice in Zimbabwe and Zambia, is less complimentary of the medical profession. However, this book was written with the wisdom of hindsight, as Cowen wrote it over twenty years after leaving these countries.

Data Analysis

The data analysis and data collection processes went hand in hand, as suggested by Glaser and Strauss (1967) and Miles and Huberman (1994). At the end of each day, I wrote up my field data into comprehensive interview notes, including reflective comments about any thoughts, observations and questions which occurred to me during the course of the interview or after, in the margins of my notes. I also noted questions which were not adequately answered in an interview. As the interviews progressed, I regularly reviewed my notes to enable me to identify gaps in the data and to assess the adequacy of data already collected. This process facilitated identification of new leads which needed to be followed up, such as issues brought up for the first time in an interview which I felt were important. As mentioned earlier, the interviews became more comprehensive as the field work progressed because of the new questions and leads that emerged. After carrying out a number of interviews with a grade of doctors, I wrote a summary of the main points raised. I completed field work after six months, convinced that I had collected enough data to portray the nature of medical autonomy among government-employed doctors at the Parirenyatwa Group of Hospitals.

Having a preliminary conceptual framework enabled me to create descriptive codes for summarizing my data. I assigned different colours to my codes and then went through each interview line by line labelling them according to the suitable code. In the process of coding, I was concerned with retaining the meaning intended in the context. For example, I identified all the statements referring to the process of diagnosing, which is an indicator of clinical autonomy, and then the different factors that affect the doctor's ability to make an independent diagnosis, such as lack of and breakdown of equipment, shortage of paramedical staff to carry out the diagnostic tests, socio-economic category of the patient (which determines whether they can pay for the tests in private institutions or not), and any institutional restrictions on the number of tests that can be carried out. Each of these factors was assigned a colour code which was highlighted whenever it appeared in the interview notes and each indicator therefore had a number of factors. After coding the diagnostic theme, I proceeded to code other indicators of clinical autonomy, which include treatment, prescription and general patient management. The need to clearly outline the indicators to enable replication has been stressed by Hammersley and Atkinson (1983:186) who argue that, 'while in no sense is it necessary or even possible to lay bare all the assumptions involved in concept-indicator linkages, it is important to make explicit and to examine those assumptions to which strong challenges can be made'.

I coded all the interviews, comprising first of all, consultants, HMOs, GMOs and registrars, junior doctors; and finally the rest of the informant interviews. I then wrote descriptive summaries on the nature of each aspect of clinical autonomy as portrayed in the interviews for the different grades of doctors and the informants separately and went through the same process of colour coding the component factors of economic autonomy and regulation of education, licensing and discipline, and then writing of summaries. The summaries were examined separately and compared against each other and any patterns and differences were noted. The process of comparing data from different respondents, or respondent triangulation, is highly recommended by Hammersley and Atkinson (1983), who point out that this performs an important task of validating the findings. The emerging portraits of the different aspects of medical autonomy tended to agree to a large extent between different grades of doctors. The analysis develops from both the informants' own understanding and my own inferences, but an attempt has been made to ensure that the respondents' views are clearly portrayed and attributed to them. The analysis is backed by quotations from respondents, which were selected for their aptness in communicating the phenomenon under discussion and for their ability to add richness to the emerging picture, as suggested by Miles and Huberman (1994).

Besides using interviews of the different groups of respondents to validate each other, the process of triangulation was extended to include both comparison and validation of data from interviews with that obtained from documents and observation. In the analysis of documents, I was more concerned with interpreting the meaning of the text, as suggested by Scott (1990) and Miles and Huberman (1994). I summarized the documents and noted the salient points and the aspect of the research for which the data was relevant. In the final analysis, the points raised in the document were used to validate points raised from another source, like an interview or observation. Documents were used as the principal source of data for the historical chapters, 3 and 4, and documents were also used extensively in obtaining data on regulation of education, licensing and discipline. These data were triangulated with data from interviews, particularly with key informants. Data obtained through observation were written up soon after the observation and the notes were then filed with the relevant aspect of the research.

Miles and Huberman (1994) suggest a number of ways of testing or confirming findings which include: checking for representativeness; checking for researcher effects; triangulating and getting feedback from respondents. In terms of representativeness, the size and level of representativeness of the sample was discussed and justified earlier in the chapter. It is almost impossible to completely eradicate researcher effects because social interaction creates behaviour in others that would not have occurred normally (Philis, 1971; Miles and Huberman, 1994). In my own research, there was little danger of my 'going native' because the group that I was researching has undergone a long process of socialization and possesses special academic qualifications which I do not possess. I did not spend enough time with them to begin to identify with them and therefore I remained very much an outsider. This could have influenced the behaviour of my respondents to an extent. For that reason, I was careful that statements describing the situation in the hospital as 'very bad' by the junior doctors were not intended to justify the strike and elicit sympathy, particularly after they were sacked and there was change of public opinion. Fortunately, their statements could be compared with those of other ranks of physicians in the same hospital who did not go on strike. Respondent validation was not carried out because of time constraints.

Problems and Ethical Dilemmas Encountered

Throughout the research I encountered a number of practical problems and ethical dilemmas, such as those of gaining access and ensuring the anonymity of my informants. Some of the ethical questions which the researcher has to contend with include: the worthiness of the research question; protecting the privacy, confidentiality and anonymity of informants; guarding against exploitation of informants; and ensuring that the findings do not harm informants (Miles and Huberman, 1994).

I have already described the hurdles I had to overcome to obtain access at the different stages in the research process. The process of negotiating access extended over the whole field work period, that is mid-January to mid-July 1994. One of the unavoidable problems which I encountered was the sudden onset of the strike which occurred before I had interviewed any of the junior doctors. Consequently, all my data reflect the respondents' feelings during and after the strike, when it would have been useful to explore their feelings before the strike, since this information would have enabled me to assess the extent to which their attitudes to government employment and strike action changed because of the strike outcome. Carrying out field work during the strike was both a blessing and a disadvantage, as the research topic became even more sensitive, which made the respondents cautious about the possible uses to which the information which they provided could be put.

In the course of field work, I was assigned a number of roles, some of which were not compatible with data collection. For instance, I was identified as nurse, student, wife, friend and researcher. During the Kadoma workshop discussed above, when I asked the chairperson about the medical audit system which he had spearheaded, he told the workshop that, 'I do not know what happened to this girl. She was a very quiet nurse and she never used to argue with anyone'. It put me in an awkward position in that he was the chairperson of the workshop and I was not exactly a legitimate participant, yet I wanted to use the opportunity to get as much information about the audit system, on which he had presented a paper at the workshop.

I also had to be careful not to offend him because I wanted an interview later.

Often I found myself cast into a culturally stereotypical gender role of married woman and was expected to behave like a respectable one who does not argue and sit with strange men. While that served to enhance my acceptance by female participants, it sometimes worked against me. At the Kadoma workshop, women participants expected me to sit with them at break times, but I wanted to take every opportunity to collect data from the various respondents, and the fact that I sometimes chose to sit with men during break time was considered aggressive. Fortunately, there were also some senior female health workers whom I interviewed in private. I was able to maintain friendly relations with women, while at the same time managing to secure extensive interviews with a number of the male participants.

My experience contradicts Golde's (1970, cited in Burgess, 1982) conclusion that mature women have the greatest scope for doing field work as they cannot be stereotyped like young single women, and a contradiction arises because of the cultural context of my research. In Zimbabwe, it is generally acceptable, though frowned upon, for a single woman to associate with men to whom she is not related but for a married woman it is unacceptable. The fact that I was a mature married woman protected me from sexual overtures during field work, so to that extent Golde's (1970, cited in Burgess, 1982) label of a married status as a protective role is valid.

The fact that I had to rely on political patronage to obtain access to carry out research posed ethical problems because of the implicit corruption inherent in such practices and the only consolation was that I did not have much subsequent contact with my patrons and did not have to register my gratitude beyond 'thank you very much'. While some of my respondents may have gained little from talking to me, others clearly appreciated the opportunity to let off steam and set the record straight to a non-judgmental audience, particularly in the aftermath of the junior doctors' strike. I promised to give senior officials in the Ministry of Health a copy of the thesis in the hope that they may gain some insight into some of the Ministry's problems.

The ethical dilemmas of protecting respondents have been well documented (cf. Punch, 1986; Lee, 1993). Some researchers have suggested disguising respondents and research sites (Barnes, 1979) in order to protect participants. I have experienced problems of disguising the identity of some of the more prominent informants, because their identities are closely linked with the positions they hold, which cannot be concealed without detracting from the information collected. I interviewed the Minister of Health, the President of HDA, ZMA, ZNA to name a few, all of whom made statements which they may not like repeated or even attributed to themselves, and yet the statements contribute significantly to the research. Often respondents told me that the information they gave me was strictly 'off the record'. I have tried to include the information without mentioning the identity of the informant. Except for the president of HDA who gave me an interview for three hours in one sitting, I saw the above mentioned respondents on two or more occasions, established some rapport and I felt that at times they forgot that they were in an interview situation, talking very freely. I have tried to leave out some of the more delicate and potentially damaging information.

Fielding (1982) has argued for dispensing with respondent anonymity in order to reduce researcher falsehood and carelessness, arguing that in the case of public personalities, they should know that whatever they say is 'on record' (Fielding, 1993). While it might be argued that this pursuit of academic excellence is commendable, I would argue against it on the grounds that even the relatively powerful respondents are sometimes vulnerable and that they deserve some consideration for their generosity. Punch contradicts Fielding and reminds researchers not to 'foul the nest' for others (Punch, 1986). I feel a particular responsibility not to close the door for local sociologists, particularly in a situation in which research access into the government health sector is given more readily to foreign researchers. When I sought access from institutions and individuals, I clearly explained that this was for a doctoral thesis and some may have relaxed their guard on the assumption that it would remain on a shelf in a British university library to which very few Zimbabweans will ever have access.

There were other minor ethical dilemmas which I encountered, particularly during the strike. One of the main complaints of the striking doctors was that they could not afford to buy cars and whenever I went to hold interviews while they were on strike, I tended to leave my car out of their view, in case it became a barrier alienating them from me. I was invariably asked whether I had a car and I had to say I had, but that it was so unreliable that sometimes I caught the bus. This made me more acceptable in the eyes of junior doctors who saw me as one of the 'disappearing middle-class'. If I took a taxi, I had to get out some distance from a meeting point because doctors were complaining about their incomes and how they could not even afford a car. On the other hand, when I had interviews in the evenings, I often had to offer transport to my informants or their visitors and while this was appreciated I was glad the car was falling apart and often needed a push before it would start.

Another minor dilemma which I encountered was persistent attempts by officials from the Ministry of Health, HDA and ZMA to discover what the other side's view was, and whether I could ask a question on their behalf, particularly during the strike. Often I was told something unpleasant about other respondents and it usually went like, 'I hope they are not your friend or relative but ...'. Even though my natural inclination was to defend them, I applied what Gans (1982:54) refers to as 'emotional handcuffs' and kept quiet in case it back-fired on me, being careful not to say anything negative about any of my respondents.

Conclusion

This chapter has portrayed my research experience and the different steps of the research process that I followed. It has described the type of information sought; the data collection methods; the process of negotiating access; the research setting; the sampling procedures; the data collection methods; data analysis and the ethical dilemmas encountered. The next three chapters present the findings of the research, starting with Chapter 5, which analyses the nature of clinical autonomy exercised by the different grades of physicians at the Parirenyatwa Group of Hospitals.

3 Development of the Health Care System and the Medical Profession under Colonialism

Introduction

The aim of this chapter is to analyze the historical development of the Zimbabwean medical profession and the health services under colonialism. Sociologists of professions have stressed the need to look at the historical and structural context in which the medical profession emerged (Johnson, 1973; Larkin, 1983, 1995; Starr, 1982). According to Johnson (1973:285) this is especially pertinent because, 'it is in their relationship to the developing colonial structure that we can begin to understand the contemporary significance of professional occupations in the new states'. This historical analysis is also intended to determine the extent to which the relationship of the medical profession and the colonial state and, consequently, the nature of medical autonomy in Southern Rhodesia was similar or different from that portrayed by Johnson (1973) in his analysis of the colonial and post-colonial states. Finally, an understanding of the history of the health services and the medical profession is crucial because the post-independence health policies were not formulated in vacuum, but were, to a large extent, a reaction to the prevailing health and medical conditions which were products of colonial health policies.

The chapter examines the provision and organization of health services for the white settlers, urban black working class, and rural-based blacks, in that order. The chapter also analyses the role of the medical profession in health care provision and policy making under colonialism. The last section discusses the last minute frenetic attempts made by the medical profession, the health insurance organizations and the state to ensure that the private health sector would survive under a black majority government.

Development of Health Services, 1890 to 1980

The history of the health care system starts with the colonization of the territory in 1890. Several attempts by missionaries and other European hunters and explorers to settle in the territory that was to become Southern Rhodesia prior to 1890 were unsuccessful due to a heavy death toll from malaria (Gelfand, 1953). When the settlers finally arrived, there were, therefore, no modern clinics or hospitals in the country.

From the time of colonization in 1890 to 1923, there was no clear health policy beyond meeting the health needs of the administration, their dependents and those of the settlers. Up to this point, the country was under the administration of a multinational corporation, the British South Africa Chartered Company, whose prime motivation was extraction of wealth rather than developing the country; it was therefore not likely to want to encumber itself with heavy long-term responsibilities. The Company did not consider itself responsible for providing the health care of indigenous people, but did so reluctantly, sporadically and rather belatedly when forced to do so by the British Colonial Office (Saints Commission, 1946; Gelfand, 1953). It was not until the passing of the Public Health Act (1925) that the role of the colonial government in health care was outlined.

The Act which emphasized the government's responsibility of preventing and controlling infectious diseases, was silent on the provision of curative services and, in the absence of a clearly articulated policy, the health care system, particularly the hospital services, developed in a haphazard and uncoordinated manner (c.f. The Public Health Act, Chapter 328:462). Webster, a long serving former Secretary for Health, explained that the government 'found itself willy nilly in the role of the main provider of hospital services, faced with the responsibility of expanding and adapting them to meet the increasing demands and changing circumstances' (Webster, 197:229). Even in the absence of a comprehensively spelt out health policy, the emerging pattern in the provision of health care reflected the racist orientation of the successive settler governments, all of which were committed to segregated health services in which the quality of health care reflected the race and socio-economic status of the recipient.

Provision of Health Services for the Settlers

In accordance with the terms of the Royal Charter signed between Cecil Rhodes's British South Africa Company and the British Crown, the former was obliged to provide medical services for all the settlers in the colony. The Royal Charter said nothing about provision of health services for indigenous people but, as will be discussed below, it soon became necessary to provide health care for those in employment. The first four settler physicians came as part of the three hundred and eighty strong Pioneer Column which colonised the territory and had the responsibility of providing medical care for the British South Africa Company administrative personnel, their dependents, and the settlers (Saints Commission, 1946; Gelfand, 1953). They were joined in 1891 by trained and untrained Dominican nuns recruited in South Africa to provide nursing services, also for the settlers.

As happened in most colonies, the health services started as a network in areas where settlers were concentrated (Gilmurray *et al*, 1979). The first hospital in the country was built by Dominican nuns in Salisbury in 1891 and thereafter, hospitals were established in the main white settlement centres, that is in Bulawayo, Gwelo, Fort Victoria, Enkeldorn, etc. By 1925 there were eleven hospitals built, staffed and financed by the Government, each run by a Surgeon-in-Charge or Medical Superintendent who looked after the administrative personnel, their dependents, prisoners and the destitute for a fixed retainer fee from the colonial administration. The doctors also looked after settlers on a fee-for-service basis (Gelfand, 1953; Webster, 1972) while nurses and all other paramedical personnel who worked in these hospitals were paid by the government. A few private nursing homes established in the first decade closed down within the decade because of financial problems, and, until 1937, when the first private hospital, St Anne's, was opened, all white patients were admitted to government hospitals which comprised both private and general wards.

A government Department of Health, headed by a Medical director, was established in 1897 and was more concerned with combating tropical diseases like malaria, bilharzia, hookworms, small pox and dysentery, to which the settlers unaccustomed to the climate succumbed in the early years (Gelfand, 1953; Cowen, 1995). As the colony became more established, the disease patterns of the settler population reflected their affluent life style and were identical to those prevalent in developed countries such as heart disease, high blood pressure and various types of cancer (Gilmurray *et al*, 1979).

The hospital facilities for the white community were described as 'adequate, even plentiful' and comparable to the best in the world (Saints Commission, 1946:20). For example, the number of general beds for whites were 70.6 per 10,000 people, compared to Great Britain's, then estimated

71

at 53.4 (Public Health Department Annual Report, 1937). The patients paid hospital fees which covered food, nursing services, drugs, diagnostic tests, surgical procedures and ward accommodation. The Saints Commission (1946:20) complained that, 'to the government the patient pays a fee which at its maximum is markedly sub-economic, but is reduced in size to a very large number of patients who come into one or other of the various concession classes'.

The health services for the white population expanded as the population multiplied naturally and through high levels of immigration from a mere 380 in 1890, to 23,606 in 1911 and 268,000 in 1977 (Department of Public Health Annual Report, 1912; Ministry of Health Annual Report, 1978). The quality of government health services continued to improve while the sub-economic hospital fees were maintained and one of the main effects of the high government subsidies on hospital fees was that it retarded the development of private hospitals which could not possibly compete with the high quality of government services without charging astronomical rates (Webster, 1973:8).

The colonial government, which wanted to attract immigrants to the colony, heavily subsidized health care to keep the costs down and to ensure that all whites had access to health facilities comparable to those in developed countries. Andrew Fleming Hospital (now Parirenyatwa) which was specifically built as a government-run private hospital and opened in 1974, compared favourably with the best hospitals in Britain of the time and yet the hospital charges only covered a third of the costs incurred, excluding the cost of the buildings and the cost of training the health workers (MOH, 1984). The patients admitted to the hospital were only attended to by private consultants or specialists on a fee-for-service basis, except for poor whites whose expenses were the government's responsibility. It is small wonder, then, that although Andrew Fleming Hospital served 8.7 per cent of the population, it consumed 29.7 per cent of the national annual health budget (Gilmurray et al, 1979:35).

In addition to government and private health services, both urban and rural local authorities provided primary care facilities such as infectious disease hospitals, dental services, and family planning facilities for the white residents. The government provided a grant to support the city health departments, but the community also contributed towards these services (Gilmurray et al, 1979).

Most of the whites resident in rural areas were large-scale commercial farmers or were engaged in mining. In the early days they were relatively disadvantaged in comparison to their urban counterparts because district surgeons charged extra for travel and productive time lost in the process. The problem was compounded by the fact that most of the settlers' economic ventures were not immediately viable and paying for health care presented serious hardship for rural whites, as Gelfand (1953: 234) points out, 'hardly a farmer's congress or a session in the Legislative Council passed without the question of the district surgeon and his high fees being discussed' (Gelfand, 1953:234). To ease the burden for them and to ensure their economic survival, in 1920 the government offered district surgeons a civil servant status with a pension, leave and a salary to remain in less lucrative areas and look after the rural based-settlers. They still treated settlers on a fee-for-service basis for those living within a ten kilometre range of the doctor's base but charged a government set travel allowance for those who lived beyond that range. The lack of viability of fee-for-service practice and the grateful reception by doctors of the civil servant status at this time, confirms Freidson's (1989) contention that solo fee-for-service does not necessarily give the physician economic autonomy.

Health insurance It is evident from the above discussion that even though health care was subsidized, settlers found paying for it on a cash basis expensive and stressful. To assuage the distress arising from this, employment organizations initiated health funds to which they and their white employees contributed fifty per cent, respectively, and these funds were administered by medical aid societies. By 1939, most of the big organizations such as Rhodesia Railways, the Public Service, Lonrho and banks had medical aid insurance schemes for their white employees.

In 1939, a larger organization, the Commercial and Industrial Medical Aid Society (CIMAS), comprising forty five smaller organizations, was formed on the same basis as above. By 1955, CIMAS had grown to include three hundred and eighty organizations and over ninety thousand members (Philip, 1956). The problem with all the medical aid societies in existence was that they did not cater for individuals and, consequently, the needs of farmers and other unorganised proprietors were still not met.

The burden of organising and providing health services motivated government to explore other ways of financing and organising health care. The colonial government appointed the Saints Commission to review the structure and functions of the health services and to propose future organization and funding of health care in the colony. The Commission consulted widely and made wide ranging recommendations in 1946,

73

including the establishment of a national health service to which all adult citizens would contribute according to ability. Everyone would be eligible for free health care once they had paid the maximum possible for their level of income. The Saints Commission reluctantly recommended that private medicine could be retained in view of the tradition established in the colony, but those who preferred it would have to pay the actual cost price for use of government hospital facilities, in addition to fees for their private practitioner. Hospital fees in government hospitals were to be increased to real cost levels to encourage the establishment of private hospitals.

Other recommendations of the Saints Commission will be discussed in the relevant sections. The establishment of a national health service was fiercely opposed by the British Medical Association and, consequently, it was not implemented. Instead, government ensured that private health insurance was attractive and affordable by making the contributions towards medical aid exempt from taxation for both the employer and the employee (Bloom, 1985). By 1980, it was estimated that the private health sector constituted over 25 per cent of the total health budget, even though that sector looked after less than 5 per cent of the total population (MOH, 1984). Government subsidy on private health care kept costs low and contributed to the boosting of demand for private medicine because it was affordable.

The establishment of health insurance was a historic landmark for the medical profession, as payment for services for patients on medical aid became guaranteed and patients were no longer deterred from consulting a doctor by lack of funds, which in turn led to an expansion of the private medical sector. The Saints Commission (1946) noted that in organizations with health insurance, there was evidence of over-visiting and excessively high rates of surgery, some of which could not be justified. There was no regulation of the rates physicians charged their patients, indeed they could ask their patients to pay for the shortfall if their charge exceeded the rate agreed with the health insurance organization (Bloom, 1985).

The lucrative nature of private medicine led to the employment of a disproportionately high number of health personnel in that sector, leaving the government sector with acute shortages, and reduced doctors' dependence on government work, particularly in its outlying hospitals. Throughout the colonial era, the private medical sector had more physicians than the government sector which served over 90 per cent of the population (Gilmurray, 1979; Saints Commission, 1946).

The provision of health services under colonialism reflected the existing political, socio-economic and racially based inequalities. While superb health services were provided for the settler community, the colonial administration in Southern Rhodesia, as elsewhere in Africa, was extremely reluctant to provide health care for blacks (Agere, 1986; Gelfand, 1953; Gilmurray *et al*, 1979).

Before colonialism, all indigenous people relied on the services of traditional healers comprising herbalists, spirit diviners, general diviners, and midwives (Chavunduka, 1986; Gelfand, 1953). Traditional healers were 'generalised wise persons' who, besides their healing functions, also acted as religious consultants, legal and political advisers, marriage and social counsellors (Chavunduka, 1986).

Provision of health care for employed blacks Africans who entered wage employment, whether in mines or urban areas, lost their natural immunity to diseases like malaria and succumbed to new ones that emerged as a result of the contact of different nationalities (Gelfand, 1953). Diseases like small pox and tuberculosis, which became major killers, were unknown in Southern Rhodesia before colonialism (Gelfand, 1953, 1976). The unnatural separation of families and the low wages caused stress and also contributed to high rates of venereal diseases, alcoholism and undernourishment (Van Onselen, 1976). The picture conforms to what occurred in other parts of Africa under colonialism (Doyal, 1976).

Confronted with these circumstances, the colonial administration had to address the issue of health care for the employed Africans, if only to stop the spread of contagious diseases to the white community. The then Medical Director of Public Health in Southern Rhodesia pointed out that, '... as we want to have a healthy white nation, we have got to tackle the infectious disease in the native. The native is the reservoir of these infectious diseases' (Fleming, cited in Gelfand, 1976).

Initially, Africans working in the urban areas were treated at the back of or outside the white hospitals but gradually, rudimentary hospitals were erected for them adjacent to white hospitals in all the major cities (Gelfand, 1953). Proper African hospitals were later built, staffed and equipped by the government, but the facilities were invariably inferior to those for the settlers in terms of the quality of buildings, equipment and staffing levels. Africans could not afford the services of private physicians, given their low wages, and were therefore attended to by government medical officers, initially for free, but later had to pay for health care at the point of treatment.

In addition to government services, urban resident Africans had access to infectious disease hospitals, primary care clinics, dental, family planning and maternity services provided by city health departments on a fee-for-service basis (Gilmurray et al, 1979). The primary care centres were the first point of contact with the health care system before urban Africans could see a doctor at a higher health institution such as the outpatient department of a big hospital.

In 1957, the two largest African central hospitals, Harare and Mpilo, were formally opened in the two major cities, Salisbury and Bulawayo. They were the ultimate referral centres for Africans throughout the country and were each located within ten kilometres from similar but more sophisticated and better resourced central hospitals for the whites. All African hospitals were staffed by full-time salaried Government Medical Officers, while the only government medical employees in the white hospitals were the Medical Superintendent and later a casualty officer to deal with emergencies (Morton Commission, 1960). Most of the consultants working in the African central hospitals did so on an honorary or sessional basis, but when the medical school was opened, the medical lecturers and their students provided additional medical care.

The colonial administration was forced by the British government to improve both living and working conditions and provide health care for Africans employed in mines, who suffered poor health and were dying in hundreds as a result of the squalid and overcrowded conditions under which they were forced to live and work. The annual death rate among the mine labourers was 150 per 1,000 and in one mine it was over 700 per 1,000 (Saints Commission, 1946:5; Van Onselen, 1976). The Public Health Department also increased its control and inspection of the mine compounds (Saints Commission, 1945).

The colonial government negotiated with the owners of industrial medical services to provide health care to Africans living in the neighbourhood who were not employed by these industries and government reimbursed the industries for this. By 1977, industrial medical services employed 36 doctors and had 10 hospitals and 18 clinics with a total of 1,379 beds (Gilmurray et al, 1979).

Farm labourers working on white-owned large-scale commercial farms (LSCF) and constituting 23 per cent of the African population, were one of the most socio-economically deprived and under-served groups in terms of health care provision (Clarke, 1977; Loewenson and Sanders, 1988). They lived under the most squalid and overcrowded conditions and lacked basic amenities like latrines and clean water. Commercial farms, comprising vast tracts of private land, were served by rural clinics, most of them were inaccessible because of the long distances from individual farms.

Health care provision for blacks in rural areas As was the typical pattern under colonialism, the administration was not interested in the welfare of Africans in the countryside who did not contribute directly to the economy. The government itself only started providing health services for rural Africans in 1931, though it had started giving missionaries an annual grant in 1927. The first missionary health services were established at the Umtali Mission in 1893. Up to 1927, health services for Africans resident in the rural areas were provided by the missionaries, but the majority relied on traditional medicine. Since Africans were reluctant to embrace Christianity, medical services and education were used to win converts and undermine traditional institutions and practices (Doyal, 1979; Gelfand, 1976). The colonial medical director summed up the missionaries' motivation for offering health services, 'medical treatment of natives is a recognised part of the missionary's work and is one of the methods adopted for attracting the natives' (Fleming, cited in Gelfand, 1976:15).

Africans in the rural areas were reluctant to use western medicine and continued to rely on traditional healers and, consequently, traditional health and cultural practices were actively discouraged and suppressed by the missionaries (Gelfand, 1976; Chavunduka, 1986). Settlers perceived traditional healers as custodians of cultural beliefs and practices which had fostered resistance and hostility to colonialism, culminating in the first indigenous rebellion of 1896-97 (Gelfand, 1976). Missionaries considered traditional religion as evil and inimical to Christian conversion, while medical professionals, who were as ethnocentric as the other settlers, considered traditional practitioners as charlatans (Chavunduka, 1986). Curtailing traditional medicine was also aimed at promoting a market for medical and pharmaceutical services (Chavunduka, 1986). The combined hostility of the missionaries, the colonial administration and the medical profession led to the passing of the Witchcraft Suppression Act (1899), which seriously curtailed the activities of traditional healers, even though a large proportion of Africans, in fact, continued to rely on traditional medicine because modern health care institutions remained inaccessible to them due to cost and distance (Chavunduka, 1978, 1986).

The colonial government was partly against funding missionary health services because, initially, most of them had no trained health care workers, most of the missionaries had taken a six-month training course in tropical diseases at the David Livingstone College in London, with the first missionary trained physician only arriving in the colony in 1925 (Gelfand, 1953). In response to pressure from the British Colonial Office in London, the government undertook to provide grants to medical missionaries employing qualified medical personnel in the rural areas in 1927. The grants were for paying the salaries of medical missionaries and nurses, maintenance of native hospitals, the establishment of training schools for native male and female nurses, the purchase of drugs and dressings and the upkeep of out-door dispensaries (Government Notice 335, 17 June 1927). The government contributed a third of the total costs of running the mission hospitals, with the rest met from hospital fees and donations from abroad (MOH, 1984:19). By 1958, there were 64 missionary run hospitals and clinics in the rural areas, providing 2,011 beds for Africans (Morton Report, 1960) and by 1977, missionaries owned 30 per cent of the total beds in the country, 66 per cent of beds in the rural areas and treated 22 per cent of the total number of outpatients (Gilmurray et al, 1979).

It was not until 1931 that the colonial government decided to provide its own rural health facilities. The country was divided into large areas and each was provided with a rural hospital surrounded by several dispensaries less than fifty miles apart (Gilmurray et al, 1979). African nurses and orderlies who provided health care at the dispensaries and rural hospitals were supervised by white nurses from the general hospitals in the main towns and a Government Medical Officer stationed at the general hospital visited the rural hospitals regularly (Webster, 1973).

As was the case in the urban areas, local authorities in the rural areas were responsible for primary care clinics providing a range of health services. These were run by the African councils, which received a 50 per cent grant-in-aid from the government for the cost of buildings and salaries of staff. By 1977, there were 363 clinics, but these were generally impoverished because rural people were not able to contribute much towards health services (Gilmurray et al, 1979).

The analysis of provision of health services under colonialism indicates a very skewed picture in favour of settlers, followed by the urban black working class, with the least of the government's concerns being the rural-based Africans, whose responsibility it readily delegated to missionaries and councils at minimum cost to itself. This was in keeping with colonial policy, which conditioned provision of health care on the capacity of the population to pay for it (Doyal, 1979). In the absence of a clearly enunciated health policy and government reluctance to provide health services for all sectors of the society, it was inevitable that the health services were uncoordinated and so grossly inequitably distributed. On the eve of independence, health services were provided by government; urban and rural local authorities; missionaries; industrial medical services; private medical practitioners and traditional healers.

The heavy emphasis on urban and curative facilities at the expense of rural and preventive services was logical, given the disease patterns of the favoured population; about 44 per cent of all health expenditure was spent on the four central hospitals in the two major cities, while the rural areas only accounted for 24 per cent (Gilmurray *et al*, 1979). Similarly, 79 per cent of doctors and 55 per cent of nurses worked in urban-based hospitals, even though 80 per cent of the population was rural-based. The government provided one bed for every 255 whites and for every 1,261 Africans (Gilmurray *et al*, 1979). The unit cost for treating a patient at Andrew Fleming was Z$42.17 (excluding the cost of medical services, which were met privately) while the unit cost at Harare hospital was Z$17.28, including medical services, as the doctors were all government employees (MOH, 1984:13). In 1979, it was estimated that there was 1 doctor for every 830 white patients, compared to 1 doctor for every 100,000 Africans in the rural areas (Gilmurray *et al*, 1979). The per capita expenditure on health services for the three groups in 1979 was Z$144 for whites, Z$31 for urban blacks and Z$4 for rural blacks (MOH, 1984:30). Almost 86.7 per cent of the health budget was spent on curative services while only 9 per cent was spent on preventive services.

The Medical Profession under Colonialism

The medical profession in Southern Rhodesia evolved with the establishment of the white settler state. It is critical to appreciate that the medical profession in Southern Rhodesia, a settler colony, differed from that in other African countries portrayed by Johnson (1972). In other African colonies, both the colonial administrators and the physicians were full-time employees of the British Colonial Office in London and carried out instructions of the Colonial Office. Their stay in any one country was only temporary and evidence suggests that they were not in any way committed to the policies which they carried out. This was certainly the case in Nyasaland (now Malawi) and Northern Rhodesia (now Zambia) (Morton Commission, 1960). The physicians in Southern Rhodesia were largely settlers, most of whom were self-employed and effectively influenced health policies through the activities of their professional association. In fact, one of them, Dr Godfrey Huggins, later Lord Malvern, rose to the level of prime minister of the colony. As will be shown below, the role of the medical profession in Southern Rhodesia was critical for the colonization process and stabilisation of the colonial state and, partly because of this, physicians were a respected and influential group. Their contributions during the colonial era were gratefully acknowledged by the colonial society,

> Readers will learn ... how tropical diseases which had defeated the original efforts of Europeans to colonise Central Africa from the sixteenth century onwards were at last conquered and brought under control. Rhodesians will realise afresh how much they owe to the devoted efforts of the first doctors and nurses. ... One of the greatest contributions that medical science has made to Southern Rhodesia ... it has sent here two remarkable doctors who have exercised a profound and beneficent influence in the realm of administration and statesmanship in the early days, Sir Starr Jameson, whose body lies beside that of his friend Cecil John Rhodes ... and Sir Godfrey Huggins to whom this book is fittingly dedicated. (Sir Kennedy, former Governor of Southern Rhodesia, in a Foreword to Gelfand, 1953:unpaged)

Most physicians who came to the colony were, like other settlers, motivated by a desire to make a better living for themselves and they were as committed to private enterprise as the other settlers were. Godfrey Huggins (later Lord Malvern), the most famous doctor in the colony, gave up an appointment at Guys Hospital in London because medical work in Southern Rhodesia paid better (Gann and Gelfand, 1964).

The colonial administration needed the services of physicians to meet the health care needs of the settlers, as prescribed by the Royal Charter, and also to make the colony an attractive destination for potential immigrants essential for the establishment of a white settler state. The medical profession, on the other hand, needed favourable health policies which would promote a viable private medical sector and this made the relationship between the state and the medical profession one of mutual dependency, with each side needing the other to meet its objectives. The social organization of health care described above and government funding of white health facilities secured them considerable economic autonomy, as will be discussed below.

A surgeon-in-charge, who was the hospital head, looked after the colonial administration employees, their dependents, prisoners, and the destitute and reported directly to the Medical Director of Southern Rhodesia. He or she was responsible for coordinating the activities of the hospital and supervising other health workers, and ensuring the safety and adequacy of drugs, medicines and instruments. He or she was paid fixed retainer fees for government duties, but had a right to look after settlers on a fee-for-service basis.

The second category of doctors were the district surgeons, who looked after the rest of the settlers on a fee-for-service basis. In the absence of a surgeon-in-charge, as was sometimes the case in small settlements, the district surgeon took over the functions of looking after government-responsibility patients for a fee. All physicians undertook some government duties, such as attending to contagious diseases and vaccinations and medico-legal work, including post-mortems and inquests, in their area. While the surgeon-in-charge was paid a fixed fee for this work, the district surgeon was paid for any government work and any medico-legal work according to government set rates on a *pro-rata* basis. When district surgeons travelled on government duty, they were paid mileage and a daily subsistence allowance (Gelfand, 1953:230).

The fees for the different medical procedures which the district surgeon carried out on government patients were clearly laid down by the administration. If a district surgeon undertook an operation on government patients or employees, they had to furnish a certificate to show that the operation was necessary (Regulations for District Surgeons, undated:7). This is comparable to some of the procedures adopted in the United States today, such as the requirement to obtain a second surgical opinion before surgical operations, instituted to reduce unnecessary procedures (Dohler, 1989; Harrison and Schulz, 1989).

Fees paid for government work were valued by district surgeons for their regularity, especially in the first two decades when physicians' incomes from private patients were not very reliable. The district surgeons' income from government work was an important control mechanism for the government, which could threaten to stop using a surgeon's services if they contravened government regulations. However, surgeons still had considerable economic autonomy as their contract could be terminated by either side with a month's notice and the British South Africa Company could not transfer them to another district without their consent (Gelfand, 1953). In their treatment of private patients, surgeons determined their own fees and their clinical performance was completely free of regulation by government and other physicians, and even when patients were admitted to government hospitals, they did not have to supply a certificate for any surgery undertaken.

Representatives of farmers and miners consistently complained to the Medical Director and to the Legislative Assembly about excessively high medical fees charged largely because of the distances which the surgeons had to travel to attend to patients in isolated areas (Gelfand, 1953). While their urban-based colleagues could refuse to attend to a patient, district surgeons had no such option because they were the only doctor in the district. In fact, even in urban areas, general practitioners were not completely autonomous from their patients because the clientele was 'politically minded' and, in addition, it was difficult for a physician in such a small community to refuse their demands (Saints Commission, 1946). Refusal to attend to a patient by a district surgeon led to an adverse report to the colonial administration and one of the consequences could be withdrawal of government work which many could ill-afford in the early days (Gelfand, 1953). Consequently, district surgeons could not choose their patients and this put them at the mercy of their patients to an extent.

The resignation of Dr Rand, a hospital-based surgeon, from the British South Africa Company in 1892 set a precedent for full-time private practice in the colony. He refused to carry out any work for the British South Africa Company after his resignation and only treated settlers privately outside the existing state institutional framework. The significance of Rand's resignation lay in that he opened up the possibility of complete private practice when the circumstances made it economically viable to do so (Gelfand, 1953). By the beginning of the twentieth century, there were general practitioners in the major settlements who relied entirely on private practice. As the market for private practice expanded in urban areas, it became increasingly difficult to attract physicians to work as district surgeons (Fleming, 1920, cited in Gelfand, 1953:236).

District surgeons were subsequently offered the position of government medical officers with civil servant status, pensionable, with leave and higher salary but, in addition, they were allowed to practise privately. This evidently provided the doctors with some economic security without removing their autonomy to earn extra income from private work. The problem was settled for the moment, but staffing of outlying stations remained a problem for the colonial government because, as the urban population increased, private practice in urban areas became more attractive and more viable. Consequently, these posts were filled by foreign physicians who came for a number of years to obtain experience before they settled down in their own countries.

Physicians and Government Hospitals

Once hospitals were established in the colony, all qualified and registered doctors could, without any limitations, admit and attend to their patients in government hospitals at any time, whether in a general or private ward. This arrangement was satisfactory when there were a few physicians, but as the population of both the patients and physicians grew, management problems emerged (Saints Commission, 1946). The Saints Commission found unlimited access disruptive to hospital routine and argued that it led to abuse of government facilities by both government medical officers and general practitioners (Saints Commission, 1946).

Nurses informed the Saints Commission of problems arising from caring for patients belonging to many different doctors with varying treatment and prescribing habits. In addition, doctors turned up at all hours of the day, making it impossible for nurses to establish a ward routine or teach the student nurses in their charge. The Commission observed that the hospital in Salisbury had in fact become 'a private nursing home for general practitioners who have no responsibility for its efficient and economical running' (Saints Commission, 1946:20). Wand and Mekie, the BMA officials from London who visited these hospitals attested to the chaotic impact of unlimited medical access, 'hospital work had become so fragmented that the routine duties of nursing and administrative staff had been greatly disturbed and it had become difficult to ensure the proper attention by the nursing staff to patients' (Wand and Mekie, 1958:178). In addition, both private and government-employed doctors used hospital facilities instead of their private rooms for consulting with their private patients. Emergency cases coming into the casualty department were often not seen promptly because government physicians were attending to their private patients (Saints Commission, 1946).

Suggestions by government to limit access to a few physicians were rejected by the local branch of the BMA on the premise that this violated the doctor-patient relationship and would affect the healing process. The Saints Commission (1946:21) complained 'What was originally conceded as a privilege has become, in the minds of some doctors, a right'. The Commission concluded that the privilege enjoyed by general practitioners in Southern Rhodesia 'obtains in the hospitals of no other government in the Empire and is only defensible so long as no better alternative is available' (Saints Commission, 1946:20). The Commission concluded that the problem could only be resolved by withdrawal of this privilege because it was being abused and was no longer in the public interest but, this was rejected by the medical profession.

Within government hospitals, physicians had almost total clinical autonomy since they were not answerable to consultants or colleagues. There were no hierarchical medical structures in the white hospitals since all, except the medical superintendent, were private practitioners. After the demise of the British South Africa Company administration in 1923, everyone except prisoners and the destitute paid for their own treatment. Each hospital had a medical superintendent but he or she was too busy and relatively powerless to sanction his or her peers, in terms of their clinical behaviour in the hospital. Some of the physicians carried out surgical operations without carrying out adequate investigations and there were suspicions that some of the surgical operations were unnecessary but intended to increase physicians' income. In addition, some operations requiring a 'high degree of skill and experience' were carried out by physicians without those qualities (Saints Commission 1946:21).

As already noted, the Saints Commission recommended the creation of a national health service and the appointment of full-time salaried physicians, including consultants, to serve in both white and black hospitals. These had to be of a high calibre so that patients admitted to hospitals could confidently submit to their medical expertise in government hospitals without worrying about the quality of service. A medical review committee was to be established to ensure that physicians did not carry out unnecessary surgical operations and that only the very well qualified performed such operations (Saints Commission, 1946). As a concession to the absence of private hospitals, and the prevailing strong tradition of private medicine in the colony, the Commission recommended that some private physicians could continue to admit their patients to government hospitals, but that the medical superintendent would have to limit the privilege of access and exercise greater control over those with access (Saints Commission, 1946). The government was advised to make the salaries more attractive and to prohibit private practice. Although government physicians would still offer private services to patients who had no access to private practitioners, the fees were to go to government and the physicians would receive an allowance for providing the service.

Some of the recommendations of the Saints Commission, such as the appointment of full- time medical staff, were only implemented in African hospitals where no private services were offered, but the medical staffing policy in hospitals for whites remained the same. Physicians in senior government positions contributed to the rejection of the national health service proposals, as pointed out at the retirement dinner hosted by the BMA for Dr Morris, the Medical Director who would have been responsible for implementing the recommendations. He was thanked for having,

> skilfully and with determination steered the profession clear of these threats ... We believe he has retained for it its freedom - and this is something which is vital to each one of us and for which the profession has to be grateful. Today ... we find the medical profession in Rhodesia in an almost unique position, for there is hardly a place in the world where the private practitioner is so well off and enjoys such status in the public eye. (Gelfand, 1958: 171)

In his response, Dr Morris pointed out that he could have done more but the medical profession had often been unclear on what it wanted, with different branches presenting conflicting views. This seems to support Bjorkman's (1989) and Wolinsky (1988) point that doctors in decision-making positions in government agencies continue to work in the interests of the profession. This is particularly applicable in the case of Southern Rhodesia, where most of the medical professionals appointed to top government positions continued to practise even as they held those positions, as in the case of Dr Blair, who practised privately for all the time that he was Medical Director of the colony, from 1897 to 1931. Almost all physicians who held senior government or administrative positions went back to private practice after retirement, making it unlikely that they would have voluntarily supported a scheme which threatened their livelihood.

In the face of stiff opposition to the proposal to limit physician access to government hospitals by the BMA, that recommendation was not implemented either (Wand and Mekie, 1958; Webster, 1973). In fact, nothing was done about the unlimited medical access to government hospitals until the Southern Rhodesia Trained Nurses Association complained to the Minister of Health about the disruptive impact of unlimited access on nurse training (Morton Commission Report, 1960). Attempts by the Minister of Health to restrict privileged access were stiffly resisted by the local branch of the BMA which argued that unlimited access to government hospitals gave private patients access to specialised diagnostic services but, more importantly, it enhanced the status of the practitioners in the eyes of their patients and hospital-based friends. The medical profession received a lot of support from the British Medical Association in London on this issue, particularly from its Chairman, who visited Southern Rhodesia in 1956 and held meetings with the Prime Minister, the Minister of Health, the Governor of the colony, several members of parliament and the superintendents of the major hospitals, and pushed the interests of Southern Rhodesia's medical profession (Wand and Mekie, 1957).

As a concession, the government appointed the Murphy Commission comprising representatives of the BMA branch in Southern Rhodesia and the Ministry of Health, and asked them to devise ways of limiting access. The Commission recommended appointment of limitation committees to determine who should have access and its recommendations were implemented in 1955 (Morton Commission Report, 1960). The limitation committees for each hospital were comprised a minimum of at least three physicians out of the six members. As it turned out, the selection process was so lax that almost everyone who applied was admitted, for example, a 183 bed hospital ended up with 86 physicians. One exasperated medical lecturer complained that, 'no less than 27 doctors visited patients between 8 am and 12 noon - an impossible state of affairs in a training school and a deterrent to the efficient running of the ward' (Levy, 1962:74).

In 1962, the Rhodesian government created a proper career medical structure in government hospitals with promotion opportunities, a salary scale, pensions, leave conditions and full civil service status. Those who accepted those conditions could no longer practise privately but would receive an allowance for providing such a service on behalf of government.

Most government medical officers in general hospitals accepted the conditions and private patients were allocated special rooms set aside for them. The new employment structure for physicians and prohibition from private practice restored the market for private practitioners which was a major victory for the BMA, which succeeded in pushing the economic interests of private medicine.

The Medical Profession and Health Policy

The discussion so far has shown that the medical profession was an important, respected and well organized group in Southern Rhodesian colonial society and was able to influence health policy to its advantage through the activities of the local branch of the BMA; by virtue of its expertise; through the activities of physicians in senior administrative positions; and by sharing the same social, economic, political and cultural values as the ruling elite.

The medical profession was able to effectively oppose some health policies through the activities of BMA local branches which actively lobbied Government and, in turn, were regularly consulted by the government on health policy. It was the local branches of the BMA which persuaded government to bestow civil service status on district surgeons in 1921, who thereafter gained pension and leave benefits while retaining their right to practise privately, thus enhancing their economic autonomy. The professional association played a major part in maintaining unlimited access to government hospitals for private physicians, thus securing further economic autonomy for them. Private physicians were able to admit their patients into government hospitals with all the facilities at reasonable prices and greatly contributed to the growth of the private health market and its stability. We noted that the BMA successfully repelled the threat posed by the establishment of a national health service.

Until 1965, the power of the medical profession derived from its links with the BMA, which lent support to its branches in the empire. A positive assessment of the quality of health services by the BMA, which was influential and respected in Britain, had the potential of boosting immigration to the colony. Until the colony produced its own medical graduates in 1968, it was entirely dependent on immigrant physicians to satisfy the health needs of the settlers and the indigenous population. Physicians considering migration to the colony were likely to consider the BMA's assessment of the conditions of service in the colony before making their decision and this made it imperative for the colonial governments to make medical practice as attractive as possible. The lobbying activities of the BMA were boosted by the fact that the colonial governments were very receptive and permeable to the influence of white lobbying organizations who 'had much more direct channels of influence than...through elections or rubbing shoulders with officials at the club. Their representative bodies '... were not only well organized and able to articulate their members' interests but [were] also brought into consultative roles' (Cliffe, 1981, cited in Herbst, 1990:20).

Physicians in positions of influence were able to push the interests of the medical profession, whether in the Legislative Assembly, where their expertise was sought when medical issues were under discussion, or in the Ministry of Health, where some of them held senior positions. One of the most influential members of the medical profession was Godfrey Huggins, who joined parliament in 1924, when the Public Health Act of 1925 was under discussion and exerted considerable influence in its formulation. He was equally influential in the debates on the Medical, Dental and Pharmacy Bill which established the Rhodesian Medical Council in 1928 (Gelfand, 1953:69). Apparently, 'the government paid a good deal of attention to what Huggins had to say in regard to such matters; he was after all their only medical expert in the House, and the good surgeon made good use of his opportunities' (Gelfand, 1953:69). His influence is evident from the dominant position which the medical profession was granted in the Rhodesia Medical Council and other health institutions.

Physicians holding senior positions in the Department of Health vetoed policies which were detrimental to the interests of the medical profession. Calls by the Saints Commission for government to sponsor black medical students were rejected by the then Medical Director, who argued that blacks should only train in health occupations which enable them to assist white physicians. In spite of the acute shortage of physicians, policy makers in the Department of Health put the interests of the profession before those of the country. For the same reasons, the government of Southern Rhodesia would not employ physicians trained in Canada and the United States until 1957 when the Ministry of Health accepted their qualifications for registration by the Rhodesia Medical Council. It is quite clear that refusal to recognise and register physicians from these countries was intended to protect the market for private practice because missionaries doctors from these countries were allowed to work in the mission hospitals but not to practise privately.

The government's ineffectiveness in controlling private doctors' access to government hospitals was partly due to the conflict of interest on the part of the policy makers who, as physicians themselves, hoped to go into private practice on retirement from government service as pointed out earlier. A national health service, with full-time salaried physicians to which most of the people had access almost free of charge, would have seriously reduced the market for private medicine and put its future at risk.

The shared social, cultural and economic values of the medical profession, the missionaries and the colonial authorities led to the curtailing of traditional medical practice through the Witchcraft Act of 1899. As discussed earlier in this chapter, each of the above groups had different motives for opposing traditional medicine, but they all shared the same ethnocentric perceptions. For that reason, traditional practitioners were denied the right to certify illness and other official business. This left the gate-keeping functions entirely to the medical profession and securely removed competition for the market with traditional healers.

A conception of the medical profession as an integral member of a minority but dominant settler community is critical in understanding its relationship with the state. Unlike colonial officials and physicians in most British colonies who carried out the interests of the colonial power, those in Southern Rhodesia were settlers themselves and formulated and implemented their own policies in accordance with their own interests. They were neither 'adventurers nor slaves of the Chartered Company' (Phimister, 1988:180, cited in Herbst, 1990:16).

After severing links with the BMA soon after Unilateral Declaration of Independence in 1965, the Rhodesia Medical Association was able to obtain concessions for itself from a government anxious to retain the support and unity of the different sections of the white community. Creating and securing a permanent market for private medicine was therefore only one of the government's many efforts to assure the whites a privileged socio-economic life style. The establishment of health insurance organizations and their exemption from taxation went a long way in expanding and stabilising the market for private medicine and securing its relative independence from the state. Thus, although there were

> ideological splits in the White population, ... they were not significant enough to generate real electoral conflict. In addition most Whites conceived of the central conflict in their country as being between Blacks

and Whites, so the numerically insignificant White population tended to unite against the perceived Black threat rather than look for divisions among themselves. (Herbst, 1990:21)

Colonial Medical Personnel Policies

The colonial policies on medical training and employment had long term effects on the post-colonial medical staff situation and when the Saints Commission suggested in 1946 that the government should sponsor some black students for medical training outside the country, Dr Askins, the then Medical Director, opposed the suggestion, arguing 'I do not think that it would be wise to adopt in Southern Rhodesia the suggestion that we should train large numbers of natives as doctors. In other words, I think we ought to have white doctors with native orderlies and native nurses under them' (Askins, quoted in Gelfand, 1976:12).

The few blacks who had trained as medical doctors had secured sponsorship privately, or paid their own way and trained in South Africa and after working a few years in government service, most went into private practice in black urban residential areas. When the medical school opened in 1963, out of the 24 students enrolled, only 4 were black (MOH, 1990). The number of black students was always very small, and in 1979 no male black students were admitted for medical training because no male student would be admitted into the university unless they had completed military service first (MOH, 1990). Most black students chose not to go to the local university, rather than serve in the colonial army. Not surprisingly, by 1980, of the 596 students who had trained as doctors in the country, only 141 or 24 per cent were blacks (MOH, 1990:75). During the colonial era, newly qualified doctors were not obliged to serve government after graduation, and 90 per cent left the country soon after or went into private practice within the country, leaving only an average of 7 per cent of the graduates worked in the public sector (MOH, 1990). Mandaza argues that this did not present the colonial governments with undue distress, as long as white children were equipped with skills to survive in or outside Rhodesia (The National Manpower Survey, 1981).

The colonial governments preferred to recruit skilled personnel from abroad than train Africans because it was feared that if they were trained to the same level as the whites, they would demand similar working conditions and this was just not acceptable. The Rhodesian Government had bought the support of the skilled white workers by assuring them a higher position in the work place than the blacks and educating blacks would have threatened the *status quo* and cost the government important support. The perennial shortage of doctors and the disrupting impact of the escalating liberation war, left most of the outlying hospitals without medical personnel in the 1970s. In 1976, the government started training clinical nurses or 'mini-doctors', a new cadre which was to be deployed to district hospitals to carry out most of the functions of doctors of diagnosing, prescribing, treatment including procedures such as the Caesarean section. This programme did not make much difference to the staffing situation because of the small numbers trained, less than ten a year nationwide every two years, and because of the lack of commitment on the part of the Ministry of Health, which had not even created a career structure for the cadre. One of the main consequences of the colonial health policies was the gross shortage of medical personnel, which continues to plague the nation to this day.

Organization of the Medical Profession

The discussion so far gives the impression that the medical profession in Southern Rhodesia was a united body but, in fact, it was fragmented along the same lines identified by Elston (1977). There were internal cleavages stemming from employment sector, status, geographical location, gender, specialisation and race. The level of autonomy which physicians exercised in their work varied with the above factors, but this will not be discussed in any detail in this thesis, which focuses on the level of autonomy in post-colonial Zimbabwe. There were often conflicts of interest which threatened the cohesion of the profession and its ability to push its overall interests, but these were masked by the BMA and subsequently the Rhodesia Medical Association, the recognised mouthpiece of the profession in negotiations with the state.

Throughout the colonial era, the majority of physicians in the country were general practitioners looking after the settler community on a fee-for-service basis (Gilmurray *et al*, 1979). Others worked as government medical officers in African hospitals, industrial medical officers in mines and agro-industrial corporations, university lecturers, medical missionaries, and bureaucrats in the Ministry of Health and its related institutions. As pointed out above, the medical association was quite active in lobbying government on behalf of its members, but not all doctors belonged to the association. Doctors based at African hospitals did not belong and mission doctors were not active either (Wand and Meckie, 1957). For a long time, the profession presented a united face but, as will become evident below, there were some underlying conflicts arising from differences of interest between specialists and general practitioners and between the two main races, blacks and whites.

Fragmentation of the medical profession due to specialisation only began to emerge in the 1950s because up to 1946, every medical practitioner was expected to provide all medical services (Gelfand, 1976). In 1946, the government announced a special allowance in recognition of surgical experience (Gelfand, 1976) but up to 1978, there was no register for specialists and anyone could practise as a specialist. The chairperson of the Council of the BMA who visited the country in 1957 found that there were equal numbers of specialists and general practitioners and that there was tension between them, leading to an attempt by specialists in one part of the country to form their own association, the Consultants and Specialists of Matebeleland.

In 1976, general practitioners formed the College of General Practitioners of Rhodesia and began pushing for the establishment of a specialist register, which was established in July 1979 by the Rhodesia Medical Council. Specialists and general practitioners agreed that those who chose to practice as specialists or consultants could only attend to patients referred by general practitioners. The College of General Practitioners assured the Rhodesia Medical Council that it was working on additional qualifications for its members so that only those who attained them were allowed to practice privately, but this was never implemented.

The medical profession under colonialism was also fragmented along racial lines, with the majority of the doctors being white. In 1960, there were less than five black doctors in the whole country, all of whom were foreign-trained, but from 1968 onwards, a small number graduated from the local medical school each year and by 1979, a total of 58 African doctors were registered with the RMC (Gilmurray *et al*, 1979). Some of them were working in government hospitals, but quite a few had left the country for further training and this trend accelerated in the late 1970s as the liberation war escalated. With the intensification of the war, most white doctors had to serve in the colonial army to preserve the colonial state. This was a significant cause of tension and division among the physicians of different races because white doctors were members of the ruling group while the black doctors were discriminated against, in spite of their qualifications. In accordance with the Group Areas Act, blacks could not live in 'whites only' residential areas nor could they work in 'whites only' hospitals. In addition, they could not undertake private practice in urban areas except in the black residential areas, unlike their white colleagues who could locate their private offices near the city centre where they were easily accessible to the public.

In 1978, black physicians formed the Zimbabwe Medical Association. Although the association was never officially recognized, its existence symbolised underlying discontent with the other two organizations, the RMA and the College of General Practitioners. As in all other sectors of Rhodesian society, there was no interaction between black and white physicians outside the work situation. The whole socio-political environment was inimical to the development of close personal relations across race barriers.

One woman physician personally described in interview the very tense and hostile atmosphere which prevailed in the late 1970s whenever a white medical student was killed while serving in the war. She mentioned that white male students were openly abusive and the situation was saved by the fact that her group had no male black students, as none had gone for national service. These racial divisions, which have persisted into the post-colonial period, have considerably weakened the ability of the profession to negotiate with government, as will be discussed in Chapter 6.

The Neo-colonial Health System

The imminence of majority rule in the late 1970s galvanised the main players in the health care arena into action. The leadership of the Rhodesia Medical Association invited the health insurance organizations, representatives of large corporations that contributed on behalf of their employees, and Government representatives to a workshop in 1978. The main objective of the workshop was to ensure

> that the status quo be maintained under any new government. That is, that private enterprise be allowed to continue as it is at the moment, with private doctors seeing patients in their rooms and then if necessary referring patients to a consultant who may then admit the patient to hospital where they will receive private treatment. This is tremendously important in order to maintain independence and free enterprise in medicine, and also in addition it is vital in order to maintain the status quo as far as medical aid societies are concerned. Should the private sector be 'abolished' by

producing 'Nationalised Health', then the position of the medical aid societies will be precarious and the whole situation will be altered. (Cohen Report, 1978:Section ii, unpaged)

A special appeal was made for the support of the proposals by the big private corporations which contribute to private medical insurance organizations and which largely determine the policies of the National Association of Medical Aid Societies (NAMAS). The workshop participants entreated, 'the future of a medically stable Zimbabwe depends on your acceptance of our solution. Commerce and industry are the vehicles through which these concepts can become a reality' (Cohen Report, 1978:6). The participants of the workshop concluded that, 'To avoid nationalisation of health services, there must be no discrimination between the races in the availability of the health services and in the benefits provided by the Medical Aid Societies' (Cohen Report, 1978:Section vi:2).

The participants predicted that nationalisation of health services would 'be repugnant to the limited number of private sector practitioners and to those who currently enjoy their services, and would almost certainly result in the exodus of both these sectors' (Cohen Report, 1978: section vii). This was the trump card of the medical profession, since private health services were largely patronised and funded by those who control the economy, and any threat to it would threaten the economic stability of the country.

The recommendations of the Cohen Report were given a shot in the arm with the passing of the Medical Services Act (1979), which outlined the operations of private health organizations and gave anyone the right to establish private hospitals and to determine admission to these facilities. The racial segregation of health facilities was removed and replaced by the 'open' and 'closed' categories, which made access to the 'open' (former white) hospitals dependent on economic status rather than on race and denied private patients access to 'closed' (former African hospitals). The Andrew Fleming (now Parirenyatwa) and the United Bulawayo Central hospitals were to continue to provide access for private practitioners and any patients who could afford to pay the going fees. Another 400 beds in the former white wings in general hospitals, i.e. those in other urban centres beside Salisbury and Bulawayo, were also reserved for private patients. Black doctors were appeased by being granted permission to practice privately wherever they wanted. Although the Government was prepared to remove the more crude racist policies, as suggested by the Cohen Committee, the essence of its health policy did not really change as is evident in *The Five-year Public Sector Investment Plan* published in 1979 (Bloom, 1985).

The Cohen Workshop demonstrated the unity of purpose and shared ideology that prevailed between the medical profession, the medical insurance corporations, the economic institutions and the settler Government. All the parties were committed to the survival of a capitalist society in which the settler community would continue to enjoy a privileged way of life. All these parties fought and supported the war against black nationalists, waged to preserve the colonial system and obviously their views did change over night. A large number of white medical doctors left Government service on the eve of independence, or soon after, for the private sector or migrated to other countries. This emigration had a serious impact on post-colonial medical personnel policies, as will be discussed in Chapter 4.

Conclusions

This chapter has analyzed the development of health services under colonialism and highlighted their fragmentation by race, provider and geographical location. It has portrayed the inequitable distribution of health services and explained that the main reason for this was that the services were provided sporadically and reluctantly by an administration which was racist and more concerned with extraction of wealth than with equitable development of all races and regions of the country.

The analysis showed that the medical profession was able to secure many concessions from the Government. In fact, the state provided the profession with shelter, which, as we will see in later chapters, enabled it to survive, grow and become strong enough to thwart threats to its survival from the post-colonial state. The successive colonial governments, which were capitalist-oriented, promoted private medicine and created an enabling environment by: giving doctors retainer fees before private practise was lucrative and viable enough; charging sub-economic hospital fees for private patients, which made private medicine affordable and a way of life for all white patients; allowing unrestricted access to government hospitals for private doctors and their patients; removing taxes on private health insurance contributions; rejecting the proposal of a national health service; curtailing the activities of traditional health practitioners and denying them gate-keeping functions; allowing private practice to government-employed doctors in and out of government hospitals; and reducing competition in the private medical sector by restricting private practice by black doctors and denying it to expatriate ones. The final act of genius was the removal of the more crude racist health policies on the eve of independence, thus forestalling widespread demands for nationalisation of private health services because the more vocal urban workers were included in the private insurance schemes.

We have seen that the medical profession in Southern Rhodesia had considerable political autonomy, which can be described as a 'medico-bureaucratic alliance', to use Larkin's (1995) term. This was achieved through the efforts of the professional associations, the BMA and the RMA, sympathetic medical bureaucrats, and government's desire to portray the country as an attractive destination for both immigrant doctors and settlers.

Even though the profession appeared united on the surface, there were, in fact, underlying conflicts emanating from specialisation and racial differences. Fragmentation along these lines led to the creation of two additional professional associations, the Zimbabwe Medical Association for black doctors and the predominantly white College of General Practitioners. As will be seen in subsequent chapters, these underlying splits became increasingly evident during the post-colonial era, seriously weakening the cohesion of the medical profession.

4 Post-colonial Health Policies: 1980 to 1994

Introduction

This chapter reviews the health policies advocated by the post-independence government which, going by experiences elsewhere, had the potential for reducing medical autonomy. The book does not examine all post-independence health policies but only focuses on those that had the potential for reducing medical autonomy, which include: introduction of free health care; legalisation of traditional medicine; review of medical education; introduction of a bonding contract for medical graduates; curtailment of private medicine; and introduction of an essential drugs list. The actual implementation and the impact of the policies are discussed in Chapters 5, 6 and 7. Finally, an analysis is made of the organisation of the medical profession in the country after 1980.

Given the ideological differences between the colonial and the majority government, it is not surprising that the latter's proposed health policies were, generally, the opposite of the colonial ones which the proponents of that system had tried to secure with the Medical Act (1979) and the 'Five year National Development Plan' of 1979. Where the colonial Government was racist, capitalist and in favour of a fragmented health service, the post-colonial Government was socialist, egalitarian and committed to a unified health service; where the colonial Government sought to relinquish its responsibility over rural health facilities and concentrate instead on large urban hospitals, the new independence government intended to concentrate on the formerly neglected rural areas, leaving the 'overdeveloped' central hospitals as they were; where the colonial Government focused on curative services, the post colonial Government was committed to preventive services with the Primary Health Care approach as the cornerstone of its health policy. Even though the medical profession was not very vocal in the first few years, there is evidence to suggest that they liaised with some white parliamentarians who challenged most of the health policies suggested by the new government. There were twenty white members of parliament in the first parliament and among these were two

97

former colonial Prime Ministers and two former Ministers of Health. It is small wonder then that there was such acrimony in the first independence parliament.

Free Health Care

One of the first initiatives which was taken by the new government to bring about equity in health was the removal of hospital fees for those earning less than the stipulated government minimum wage of Z$150 per month. This measure was adopted in September 1980, four months after the attainment of independence and was ecstatically received by the majority of the population who fell into this category (Loewenson, 1988), estimated to be 90 percent of the population (World Bank Report, 1992). This policy was not well received by the white members in parliament who asked how the deserving members of society were to be identified and where the money was going to come from since 'free health' had to be paid for by someone. The then Minister of Health argued that if someone was black they were almost definitely deserving because the majority earned less than the stipulated minimum wage. In spite of the acrimony, the policy was adopted and implemented since the ruling party, ZANU (PF), had a large majority and the black opposition members of parliament also supported the bill.

Prior to September 1980, there was a charge for most curative services and hospital fees were determined on a sliding scale according to the patient's income, but even poor blacks sometimes consulted private medical practitioners when the health workers at the local health centre did not refer them to a doctor, or if they felt that the condition needed urgent attention. The general belief of many Zimbabwean people that proper treatment should include an injection encouraged even poor people to consult a private doctor even where the local clinic could have sufficed. I assumed that with free health care, more people would have visited the government hospitals rather than private practitioners, but no research has been carried out on the impact of free health care on the private medical sector. It is likely, though, that the number of poor people consulting private practitioners decreased but this was not so obvious because the inclusion of employed blacks in the private health insurance schemes considerably expanded the market for private medicine. However, there is evidence suggesting that more people went straight to central hospitals where they were likely to be seen by the doctor and to be given medicines, without first going to the local health centre. Enforcement of government regulations, such as attending only to those who followed proper referral channels and requiring pay slips to prove eligibility for free health care, was perceived as unpatriotic and synonymous with betrayal of the revolution, particularly in the early euphoric years. Not surprisingly, the number of patients visiting health centres increased dramatically and the large hospitals were soon overcrowded because a lot of the people who came to the big hospitals did not need, to as their conditions were not serious enough. In addition, a lot of people who were really supposed to pay for health care did not do so (World Bank, 1992) and consequently, it was not long before the hospitals were short of drugs and other essential health resources (World Bank, 1992). To make matters worse, most white patients no longer attended Parirenyatwa Hospital, preferring the elite private hospitals, thus further depriving the hospitals of badly needed funds. By the late 1980s, it had become evident that the free health system was not viable and could not be sustained much longer (World Bank, 1992).

Repeal of the Medical Services Act (1979)

The new government's commitment to formal desegregation and egalitarianism of health services was partly realised in 1981, with the repeal of the Medical Services Act (1979), giving access to anyone, including non-paying patients, to former 'whites only' hospitals. As mentioned in Chapter 2, prior to independence, patients coming to the Parirenyatwa Group of Hospitals were attended to by their private consultants and the hospitals had no medical staff establishment up to 1981, except for the medical superintendent and a couple of casualty officers to look after emergency cases and government responsibility patients. The desegregation of the hospitals made it difficult for non-paying patients to attend the hospital because they did not have personal physicians to attend to them. Government was only able to employ a few consultants because of a gross shortage in the country, as most of the white doctors had either left the country or gone into private practice and the few government consultants could not adequately deal with the huge influx of patients to Andrew Fleming Hospital in particular.

The Salisbury Hospitals Act (1975) was amended in 1981 and the Andrew Fleming Hospital was renamed Parirenyatwa Hospital, while the whole Salisbury group became known as the Parirenyatwa Group of

Hospitals. More importantly, junior doctors were allowed to work at the Parirenyatwa Group of Hospitals under the supervision of government-employed consultants and medical lecturers, as had been the case at Harare Hospital all along. A system of shared posts, whereby a doctor holds the same post at Harare and Parirenyatwa Hospital was introduced, which meant that a doctor working in orthopaedics at Harare Hospital would perform the same duties in orthopaedic wards at Parirenyatwa Hospital. Harare Hospital always had a medical staff establishment with proper hierarchical structures because it had always been a teaching hospital, with all the patients treated by government doctors and university lecturers.

The medical staff establishments for the central hospitals have not been reviewed since 1980 and, in addition to the perennial shortage of physicians in all the hospitals, this has given rise to problems of controlling the doctors on shared posts who can claim to be at either of the hospitals when they are at neither, as will be discussed in more detail in Chapters 6 and 7. Surprisingly, no medical staffing changes were instituted at Mbuya Nehanda, the best government maternity hospital which is part of the Parirenyatwa Group Hospitals, and as a result, 95 percent of the patients coming into the hospital continued to be admitted by their private consultants until 1995.

Legalisation of Traditional Medical Services

As mentioned in Chapter 2, traditional medicine was suppressed under colonialism, even though it remained popular among the indigenous people (Chavunduka, 1978). The new government recognised traditional medicine and advised the healers to form a single traditional healers' association which could negotiate with government and subsequently, the Zimbabwe National Traditional Healers' Association (ZINATHA), which had already been in existence for some time, was formally recognised in 1981 through the Traditional Medical Practitioners' Act. This Act provided for the creation of a Traditional Medical Practitioners' Council responsible for regulating the healers registered with it (Chavunduka, 1986) and from then on, it became illegal for a traditional healer to practise without formal registration with the Council. Going by the experience of the reaction of the medical profession in other countries to the recognition and registration of alternative healers (Larkin, 1983; Saks, 1995), I assumed that the medical profession would have been hostile, and that recognition would have a negative effect on the economic autonomy of the medical profession, an issue which will be taken up in Chapter 6.

The Private Medical Sector

The government expressed its opposition to the private medical sector which, it alleged was incompatible with government's cardinal principle of 'equity in health', was subsidised by the public sector, gave rise to maldistribution of health institutions and personnel, and inculcated the 'wrong attitudes' to young Zimbabwean medical graduates (Ushewokunze, 1984; MOH, 1984).

The government felt that equality in the provision of and access to health care could not be achieved as long as some members of society had access to superior private health facilities. The new Minister of Health explained that the government was committed to integration of health services, but that this was technically not possible if there was an independent private health service. The new government was also hostile to the private medical sector because it was heavily subsidised by the public sector in a number of ways. Firstly, private patients admitted to government hospitals only paid a third of the actual cost of hospitalisation at the Parirenyatwa Group of Hospitals (MOH, 1984) and secondly, private health insurance schemes, which paid for the health care of most of the private patients, were 100 percent tax-rebatable for both the employer and the employee (MOH, 1984; Bloom, 1985). This meant that those who could most afford to pay for health care were paying very little for it and, even though the then Minister of Health advised the Minister of Economic Planning and Development to remove the tax rebate, this was not done.

Initially, the government announced its intention to ban the use of government beds for private patients, but later decided that the money so obtained would be useful in the maintenance of the large urban hospitals since it intended to spend more of its financial resources on formerly neglected rural health institutions (MOH, 1984; Ushewokunze, 1984). At the same time, it refused to allow construction of private hospitals in the country, arguing that there were sufficient beds to meet the needs of private patients in both private and government hospitals. The Minister of Health alleged that the proposed hospitals intended to import the latest medical technological equipment, thus using up scarce foreign currency on a few patients. In addition, the proposed hospitals were all going to be located in the two largest cities, and this would 'accentuate the present gross maldistribution' of health institutions in favour of the already over provided urban areas (Ushewokunze, 1984:157). The proposed institutions would also syphon health workers from the already short-staffed government hospitals, which could not match the salaries and conditions of service offered by the private health sector. Furthermore, expansion of the lucrative private sector would lure newly trained medical graduates to join the private sector rather than work for government, particularly in the rural areas where they were most needed. The government announced that doctors employed in its institutions were not allowed to practise privately, even during their free time (MOH, 1984). Implementation of the above policies had a potential of seriously curtailing physicians' economic autonomy.

Review of Medical Education

In 1980, the Minister of Health complained about the small medical school intake and asked the University of Zimbabwe to double it and in 1981, the student intake was increased, from an annual average of forty, to eighty students. The Minister of Health also expressed the government's dissatisfaction with the calibre of the medical graduates produced using the old University of Birmingham curriculum which was characterised as unsuitable for training medical graduates capable of dealing with medical conditions prevalent in a Third World country (Ushewokunze, 1984). The Minister hired a consultant, Professor Nonholi, a renowned specialist on medical education working for the World Health Organisation, to review the medical curriculum and medical education in Zimbabwe. One of the recommendations made in the Nonholi Report was to increase the period of rural attachment for medical students during their training and their lecturers had to go to the field rather than leaving them to be supervised by district medical officers who were not always qualified to do so. In addition, the medical students were to be taught some behavioural science courses. The government also felt that a one year internship was inadequate to equip a medical graduate with all the skills necessary to work on their own whether in the rural hospitals or in solo private practice, and accordingly, the period of internship was increased to two years starting in 1987.

The Bonding Employment Contract

The Government's intention to introduce a bonding contract was announced in its first white paper on health in 1984, but little was mentioned about it until 1987 when the Medical Dental and Allied Professions Act was amended making it compulsory for all Zimbabwean medical graduates to work at government designated institutions for seven years after graduation, starting from 1988. The principal aim of this policy was both to increase the number of physicians in government hospitals, and to ensure that they did not join the private medical sector before they had gained sufficient experience under supervision in government hospitals. This policy, which had wide ranging implications, was received with hostility by most sections of the medical profession, but most of all by the junior doctors and those still in training.

The Essential Drugs List of Zimbabwe (EDLIZ)

In 1985, the Ministry of Health appointed a National Drug and Therapeutics Policy Advisory Committee to establish a pharmaceutical policy for the country, as advised by the World Health Organisation. The idea was to rationalise drug procurement and prescription in accordance with the country's limited resources. At this particular time, there was a critical shortage of drugs in government hospitals, coupled with a serious shortage of foreign currency reserves necessary for importing the drugs. Pharmaceutical companies such as Pfeizer, Geddes, Ciber Geigy and CAPS were inefficiently using scarce foreign currency reserves by importing a wide variety of drugs, many of them basically the same but using different trade names reflecting the multiplicity of producers. The Deputy Director of Pharmaceutical Services explained in interview that paracetamol, paramol, panadol and panado are all basically one drug, the only variation being either the taste, colour or shape of the tablets. In addition, those drugs which used trade names tended to be expensive.

The Government decided to limit the number of drugs on the market and thus conserve scarce foreign currency and, at the same time, all drugs it purchased had to use generic names. Accordingly, the committee drew up a list, known as the Essential Drugs List of Zimbabwe (EDLIZ), for treatment of the majority of diseases prevalent in the country, with the idea of limiting the variety of drugs necessary for each condition, which in turn

103

would facilitate bulk buying and effect economies of scale. Different and suitable drug lists were drawn for the different levels of health institutions in the country, starting from those that can be prescribed at simple rural health centres; through those that can be prescribed at rural, district, and provincial hospitals; to those that can be prescribed at central hospitals and others by specialists only. The EDLIZ, was first published in 1985 and revised in 1989 and 1994 respectively, outlines the common diseases in the country, their presenting symptoms, the tests necessary and suggests the management programme, including up to five drugs that can be used for the various conditions, and also outlines clear treatment guidelines and optimal dosages.

I had surmised that this policy would not only reduce physicians' clinical autonomy, but also perceived it as a potential source of conflict between government and the medical profession used to prescribing whatever they considered most appropriate. The experience of Britain on the introduction of its limited drug list in 1985 (Elston, 1991; Klein, 1989) led to expectations of similar resistance by the medical profession in Zimbabwe.

An Assessment of Post-independence Achievements, 1980 to 1989

On coming to power, the first Zimbabwean government expressed its commitment to integrating and unifying the fragmented health services which made administration and equitable distribution of health resources difficult, if not impossible, largely due to its acceptance of a dual health system consisting of, that is; public and private health sectors (MOH, 1984; Bloom, 1985; Manga, 1988). The existence of private medicine precluded achievement of equity in health because some had access to superior private health facilities.

The government managed to vertically and horizontally integrate most of the public health services which had previously been uncoordinated, including rural health services, urban municipal services, government hospitals and other public health institutions (MOH & CW, 1990). Curative and preventive health services, which were previously run independently of each other, were successfully integrated (MOH & CW, 1990). There was a notable increase in the number of health training institutions built and the number and variety of health personnel trained, although some health professions remained in short supply. However, the health system was still characterised by considerable maldistribution of health resources, including most categories of health personnel, in favour of urban institutions (Public Service Review Commission, 1989).

The achievements of the post-independence government in health care provision have almost universally been described as impressive (Loewenson, 1988, 1991; Mandaza, 1986; Sanders, 1990; World Bank, 1992). A World Bank team which was invited by the Government to help assess health services and work out strategies of financing health care in the face of rising fiscal constraints concluded,

> Zimbabwe's achievements in health during the 1980s have been truly impressive. More than 500 health centres have been built or upgraded and more than a dozen district hospitals have been completed or are under construction... All of these current indicators are significantly better than the averages of sub-Saharan Africa. (World Bank, 1992:x)

Other achievements of the post-independence government include: reduction of the infant mortality rate from 120-140 per 1,000 at independence to 70 per 1,000; very large increase in the rate of immunisation of children against major killer diseases, from 25 to 70 percent by 1989 (MOH & CW, 1990:ii) and significant expansion of family planning services and their use, expanded considerably giving the country the highest rate of contraceptive use in sub-Saharan Africa (Sanders, 1990). The expenditure on preventive services rose considerably from 10 percent before independence to 28 percent of the annual health budget and most of it was spent on rural-based projects (World Bank, 1992:39). Although health expenditure in the rural areas increased considerably, and construction at central hospitals was halted in the first few years of independence, patterns still showed an urban, high technology bias (World Bank, 1992).

In 1987, the public sector was responsible for 63 percent of all health related expenditures, private doctors, 25 percent; the industrial medical sector, 8 percent; and non-governmental organisations, 4 per cent (World Bank, 1992:x) with only 12 percent of government expenditure on health care coming from foreign aid. Public spending on health was at its highest in the early 1980s, but slowed markedly towards the end of that decade because of severe fiscal constraints faced by the government (World Bank, 1992:xi). By the late 1980s, the Zimbabwe government was facing serious economic problems, with an annual inflation rate of 25 percent (GOZ, 1991); a budget deficit of 10 percent of the Gross Domestic Product (Chakaodza, 1993); and rising unemployment levels. By the late 1980s, it had become apparent that government spending on health services was not likely to increase and that the 5 percent of Gross National Product allocated for health was inadequate to sustain the health programmes started since independence (World Bank, 1992).

An assessment of the cost recovery mechanisms, such as collection of hospital fees at government hospitals, found them weak and largely ineffective. Mechanisms for establishing patients' capacity to pay for health care were almost non-existent and, not surprisingly, a lot of people who could afford to pay hospital fees did not do so (World Bank, 1992). All the health charges were set at too low a level in relation to actual cost of services and people's capacity to pay and, consequently, those who paid were undercharged (World Bank, 1992).

There was ample evidence indicating that poor collection of user fees at central hospitals was largely due to a grossly inefficient billing system with hospital bills often not sent until 9 to 12 months after treatment, at which point most health insurance organisations were not willing to honour them since their policy is that all bills should be submitted within three months of treatment (World Bank, 1992). The inefficient collection of hospital fees seriously reduced government revenue and finance capacity (World Bank, 1992). As mentioned earlier, inefficient hospital fees collection at central hospitals rendered the patient referral system ineffective, as patients by-passed the lower but more appropriate health institutions where fees collection was more effective than at the higher ones. Health care provided at higher institutions was obviously more costly than would have been the case at lower institutions and the result was that the central hospitals were grossly overcrowded and all the health resources were soon over-stretched. The World Bank team made several suggestions, most of which were incorporated into the Economic Adjustment Programme.

Zimbabwe's Health Services in the 1990s

The World Bank and International Monetary Fund-inspired ESAP programme was officially launched in mid-1990 and implemented gradually in the different sectors of the economy (Chakaodza, 1993). Implementation of ESAP in the health sector entailed removal of subsidies and provision of all health care at cost to the consumer and accordingly, all user fees at government, mission and local authority health facilities were revised upwards in January 1994. User fees were set according to the level of the institution, i.e. fees for the Parirenyatwa Group of Hospitals' outpatients

106

were pegged much higher than those for lower health centres such as urban municipal clinics. The maximum threshold for non-payment of hospital fees was raised from Z$150 per month to Z$400 and the Ministry of Health identified mechanisms for determining the patients' socio-economic status. The World Bank's recommendation that excessive drug prescribing could be curbed by billing the patient for each drug prescribed rather than the whole prescription was implemented for paying patients (World Bank, 1992).

Another impact of the introduction of ESAP was that the Ministry of Health, like other government departments, had to reduce its health staff establishment. Where nurses were previously assured of a government job on completion of training, the situation changed after the introduction of ESAP and for the first time, some health professionals, including nurses, found themselves unemployed and many began leaving for neighbouring countries where there were better opportunities. This was in spite of the fact that most major health institutions were complaining of staff shortages (Lennock, 1994).

Meanwhile, a Social Dimensions of Adjustment Fund (SDF) was established to meet the needs of those falling below the monthly income threshold of Z$400. Since the introduction of the health reforms, government policy is that all health services have to be paid for, either by the individual, their medical insurance or the Social Dimensions of Adjustment Fund. Setting the user fees according to the level of the institution forces patients to follow the referral system because those who disregard the system and turn up at higher level health institutions are charged the fees applicable there irrespective of their level of income except in emergencies.

The increase in and stringent collection of hospital fees started in 1991 and refined in 1994 created four economically based categories of patients. Table 4.1 below shows that patients admitted to Parirenyatwa hospital now fall into four distinct categories and the quality and amount of treatment which they receive varies with the category, as will become evident in Chapter 5.

As illustrated below, the first categories are patients with a monthly income of less than Z$400 whose hospital fees are paid by the Social Dimension Fund; the second category comprises patients with a monthly income of more than Z$400 but without health insurance who have to meet medical expenses in cash out of their pocket; the third category comprises patients covered by a general health insurance policy (known as medical aid); the fourth category of patients are the well-to-do who opt for a private patient status, may have an expensive health insurance policy or may pay cash out of pocket.

At Parirenyatwa, the first three categories of patients are treated in a general ward and receive the same nursing care, food, bedding and sanitary facilities, while private patients are treated on a separate 'D' floor which offers five star hotel services where patients are tended by a much higher proportion of nursing staff than on the general wards.

Table 4.1   Categories of Patients at Parirenyatwa Group of Hospitals, 1994

	Patient Economic Status			
	Under Z$400 per month	Over Z$400 per month	Health Insurance	Private Patients
Proportion	44%	35%*		21%
Type of Ward	general	general	general	'D' wing
Payment of Fees	SDF/free	cash	health insurance	cash/health insurance
Diagnostic Tests & Treatment	doctor's discretion & availability	cost conscious	doctor's discretion	doctor's discretion

*   Combined figure for health insurance and cash-paying patients with monthly incomes over Z$400 admitted to the Parirenyatwa Group of Hospitals.

SDF, or 'free', and paying patients who are not on medical aid receive the same level of medical services from government doctors and they do not have to pay doctors' fees separately. Private patients and some of those on health insurance, on the other hand, are attended to by private doctors who may be government or university employed or private consultants. They pay the doctor separately and privately for the services rendered and, consequently, they tend to expect and receive more medical attention than SDF and paying patients without health insurance. Those on general health insurance may choose to be attended to by a Government doctor to ensure

108

that they do not incur a shortfall for which they have to pay out of pocket and, in that case, receive the same medical attention as SDF patients.

A report by the Zimbabwe Congress of trade Unions indicates that 71 percent of the workforce has difficulty meeting health costs (cited in the *Southern African Economist*, Vol. 7, No. 4, 1994). This is quite understandable because, even though some may earn over Z$400 per month, they may have large families all of whom have to pay for health care from hat amount. In 1995, the government abolished user fees in the rural areas after realising that the method of proving eligibility was too onerous and prejudiced patients' access to health care (MOH & CW, 1995). The Ministry of Health and Child Welfare is currently considering decentralising the management of health services to the newly created Rural District Councils as part of the current public sector reforms (MOH & CW, 1995) but since the policy has not yet been implemented, it is difficult to surmise its likely implications.

The ESAP and the severe drought which crippled the Zimbabwean economy in 1991/92 and 1994/95 have eroded some of the government's achievements in the health sector (MOH & CW, 1995). Its inability to cut public spending to the extent demanded by the international finance institutions has resulted in its loans being temporarily suspended and government ministries being allocated budgets on a monthly basis as from mid-1995. The budget of the Ministry of Health has been cut by 39 percent since 1990 and its financial woes are much worse because of inflation and the devaluation of the Zimbabwe dollar since the introduction of ESAP (*Herald*, 3 February 1996:1). Consequently, budgets for most hospitals have been drastically reduced, giving rise to shortages of drugs, ill-maintained equipment, shortage of intensive care beds and of blood for transfusion. At Harare Maternity Hospital, the busiest in the country, the ultrasound scan and the carditocograph, which are essential for monitoring foetal well-being, were out of order for much of 1993, making it extremely difficult for doctors to diagnose and manage patients, all of whom are referred to the hospital because they show signs of complications. It is therefore not surprising that 69 percent of maternal deaths were attributed to institutional failures (Lennock, 1994; Comptroller and Auditor General, 1995). Another example of the impact of the slashed health budget is that of Gweru Provincial Hospital whose budget was cut by more than 50 percent, leading to scaling down of services in all departments. The medical superintendent of the hospital explained that the X-ray department had reduced its services from about 60 to 20 patients a day (*Herald*, 3 February 1996:1). The shortage of funds was so drastic that in late 1995, the Ministry of Health was unable to pay its debts for food, electricity, water and drug supplies and some of the suppliers subsequently stopped supplying government hospitals. Consequently, between November 1995 and January 1996, a number of hospitals, including Gweru Provincial and Mpilo Central Hospitals, ran short of food and had to ask patients to supply their own. The state President authorised that the Ministry of Health be given a hundred million Zimbabwe dollars to pay off some of the more pressing debts after a personal appeal from the Minister of Health and Child Welfare (*Herald*, 25 January 1996:1). This pathetic state of of health services is prevalent in other African countries. For example, one of the main daily newspapers in Kenya, the *Daily Nation*, (11 June 1996:6) described the state of the Kenyan health sector as follows,

> The lack of even the simplest pain killer in some health centres and the virtual collapse of service in some major hospitals are the grim indicators of the health sector all over the country. In some areas, patients have to take with them paper on which doctors write their diagnosis and prescriptions. Congestion has forced patients to share beds (sometimes three in a bed) on bedding brought from home ... As for food forget it!

Organisation of the Medical Profession

The fragmentation of medical profession by employment sector, role, rank in the professional hierarchy, speciality, gender, race and country of origin remains in post-colonial Zimbabwe and, in fact, the number of professional associations has increased. The variety of employment sectors remains very much as described in Chapter 3, but the proportion of doctors working for the Ministry of Health is much higher than before because all government hospitals, with the exception of Mbuya Nehanda Maternity Hospital, have a medical staff establishment and hierarchical medical firm structures. Most of the top civil service posts in the Ministry of Health and Child Welfare are occupied by black doctors, as are most of the lecturing and government consultant posts. Most Zimbabwean white doctors left the public sector either just before or soon after independence in 1980, except for some employed as lecturers in the medical school. The white doctors employed in government hospitals are expatriates. The private sector, on the other hand, is dominated by white physicians, although the number of black doctors in private practise has risen considerably since the late 1980s.

110

Almost all the senior bureaucratic and consultant posts in the Ministry of Health are still occupied by male doctors. Most women doctors leave government service and work as solo fee-for-service general practitioners, which is more compatible with their family responsibilities. A comparable situation obtains in Britain, although the proportion of women in senior positions is much higher (Doyal, 1994) than in Zimbabwe where one of the medical superintendents of the central and provincial hospitals is a woman and only one woman doctor occupies a senior position in the Ministry of Health.

The shortage of physicians in the country forced government to recruit expatriate doctors and these form a distinct group from the Zimbabwean doctors. The government relies heavily on foreign expatriate doctors particularly for its outlying hospitals and for the registrar posts in all its hospitals. In addition, the employment contract for expatriate doctors prohibits them from taking part in strikes and other industrial action: this weakens the bargaining position of the local doctors while at the same time widening the gulf between the two groups as we will see in Chapter 6.

Even though the medical profession in post-colonial Zimbabwe is not more segmented than its colonial predecessor, the cleavages appear more visible than before. In 1981, the Zimbabwe Medical Association, and the Rhodesia Medical Association amalgamated to become the Zimbabwe Medical Association (ZMA) at the urging of the then Minister of Health, who stated that he was not going to talk to two different organisations of the same profession. The stated objectives of the organisation are, 'to maintain the honour and interests of the medical profession in Zimbabwe... To oppose any proceedings or applications which may seem calculated directly or indirectly to prejudice the interests of the Association' (Zimbabwe Medical Association Constitution, undated:1).

Since its inception, about 50 percent of the doctors in the country are members of ZMA although its activities appear to have been dominated by consultants. Its large membership is a result of its success in negotiating for lower insurance subscriptions with the Medical Defence Union (UK), through which almost all doctors are insured.

The College of Primary Care Physicians (CPCP), formerly known as the College of General Practice in Rhodesia, was established in January 1976 (*CAJM*, February 1976:32). The CPCP has remained largely white, although, for the first time in its history it has had a black President for the last three years. One of the reasons why black physicians have not been eager to join the organisation is its insistence after independence that new members should sit an examination. Black doctors feel that this rule was instituted on racial grounds because all the white members who belong to the organisation did not sit the examination when they joined. They also question the rationale for sitting an examination for an organisation which has no credentials recognised by the Health Professions Council. Moreover black doctors have also questioned the academic ability of those who are supposed to examine them since most have been working in the private sector for a long time dealing only with minor illnesses. Given that there is no obvious benefit for members of CPCP, most black doctors who have gone into private practice are not members of the organisation. The current president has pleaded with the other members of the organisation to waive the examination requirements until the qualifications proposed for those joining the private medical sector are recognised by the Health Professions Council, but it appears that to date he has not been successful.

The Hospital Doctors Association (HDA), which is supposed to represent all doctors working in Government hospitals, was formed in 1986 as a response to what was alleged to be the ineffectiveness of the Zimbabwe Medical Association in improving their working conditions. Although the organisation is supposed to be for all hospital-based doctors, it has largely been associated with junior doctors, i.e. interns (SRMO and JRMO) and senior house officers. This is the organisation which has had the most conflict with Government because its members are the ones most directly affected by some of the Government policies in the health sector.

The divisions within the Zimbabwean medical profession have considerably weakened the medical profession, particularly in negotiations with the government. The significance that this has for the degree of clinical, economic and political autonomy which the different segments of the medical profession exercises will be discussed in Chapter 6.

Conclusion

Some of the policies introduced by the post-independence government which include introduction of free health care; legalisation of traditional medicine; the review of medical education; the introduction of a bonding contract; the curtailment of the private health care; and the introduction of an essential drugs list, had the potential of reducing some dimensions of medical autonomy. These policies highlighted the ideological differences between the colonial and the post-colonial governments, but it remains to be seen whether they had the effect envisaged by the Government. The introduction of ESAP has reversed some of the gains made during the first decade of independence particularly universal, particularly access to health care regardless of the economic status of patients. The reduction of the health budget is also likely to have an impact on the clinical autonomy of the medical profession. Chapters 5, 6, and 7 will indicate whether there has been an erosion of medical autonomy, or whether the medical profession in Zimbabwe, like its counterparts in the United States and Britain has engaged some defensive tactics to deflect and limit this.

5 Clinical Autonomy

Introduction

This chapter analyzes the nature and extent of clinical autonomy that doctors employed at the Parirenyatwa Group of Hospitals exercise in their day to day work, including comparison of the degree to which it approximates that depicted by Freidson in his medical dominance model (Freidson, 1988, [1970]) and that exercised by doctors in the United States and Britain. Particular attention will be paid to determining the extent to which post-independence health care policies and the wider social, economic, political and cultural environment have affected doctors' clinical autonomy at the Parirenyatwa Group of Hospitals.

As pointed out in Chapter 1, there is now a general consensus among theorists writing on professions that medical autonomy is on the decline in developed countries due to challenges from: more authoritative management intent on controlling both costs and the quality of medical work through processes such as second surgical opinion, diagnostic related groups and medical audit (Light, 1991, 1993; Dent, 1995; Hunter, 1994); litigious and assertive consumers and self-help groups (Haug, 1988; Rosenthal, 1987; Kelleher, 1994); other occupations in the health care division of labour (Witz, 1994); and from alternative health practitioners (Saks, 1995). Dohler (1989) argues that increasing awareness of the limitations of medical intervention and iatrogenesis have meant that clinical autonomy is no longer sacrosanct and has exposed doctors to more economic constraints than ever before. However, there is no agreement on the degree of erosion and the likely outcome of the process, largely because the medical profession has been fighting back, either by reducing the impact of the regulatory policies or by turning them to its benefit (Dohler, 1989; Freidson, 1989, 1994; Hafferty and Light, 1995; Hafferty and McKinlay, 1993).

Doctors' Autonomy in Diagnosing

The choice of diagnostic procedures which government-employed doctors in Zimbabwe can carry out is determined by the condition of the patient, the availability of the necessary diagnostic equipment, the competence of the relevant paramedical departments to provide the services required and, to some extent, the socio-economic status or category of the patient. There are no strict administrative restrictions on choice or quantity of diagnostic tests that can be carried out within the Parirenyatwa Group of Hospitals, so physicians can to a large extend, carry out whatever diagnostic tests they consider essential for the condition of the patient.

All levels of doctors who were interviewed explained that even though there are no administrative regulations, they are often not able to carry out essential tests such as CAT scans, barium meals and some blood tests because of problems in the paramedical departments responsible for carrying out the tests. The most common problems are unavailability or breakdown of essential equipment, and a shortage of personnel to carry out the tests, both of which clearly compromise physicians' ability to accurately diagnose some medical conditions. For example, ordinary x-rays are often inadequate and a CAT scan, which greatly enhances diagnostic skills, is only available at one private health institution in the whole country. Not surprisingly, all the doctors expressed frustration with the unavailability of such essential equipment,

> the ultra-sound machine is not available, CAT scans are non-existent in public hospitals. You have to apply to the Medical Superintendent for permission to send a patient to a private one. We have problems with back-up services. Patients are not getting the best. If the patients here knew about litigation, the doctors could be sued for not using some of the diagnostic tests. (SRMO, Department of Medicine)

Doctors explained that when necessary diagnostic procedures cannot be carried out at Parirenyatwa Hospital, they can refer a patient to private health facilities, but that this is only applicable to those who can afford to pay cash for the service. Consequently, private patients are able to pay for use of private diagnostic services while other patients, including some of those on health insurance, are often not able to raise the necessary cash even though they are refunded the money by the insurance company after the final hospital bill is submitted. Paying patients whose salaries are just above the threshold of Z$400 per month and 'non-paying' or SDF patients are usually unable to raise the high fees charged for private facilities and, consequently, most cannot use such facilities. Parirenyatwa Hospital is able to fund a small number of SDF patients for the use of private diagnostic equipment but the decision as to which few get access is made by the Medical Superintendent to whom all physicians with patients needing to use the equipment must submit case files. Thus, when the need to use private facilities for SDF patients arises, the autonomy of all levels of doctors in diagnosing is transferred to the Medical Superintendent who makes the final decisions.

Inability to carry out essential diagnostic tests does not only arise from unavailability of machinery, since even when new equipment is procured, it is often not the most efficient and sophisticated available on the market, as the doctors pointed out. One example cited was that of syringes ordered from China which were allegedly crude and ineffective and were later thrown away. One consultant surgeon complained that 'new equipment is hard to come by. Procurement and management of equipment is left to autocratic despots [hospital management] who have no clue about it'. On the other hand, the Health Services Administrator of the Parirenyatwa Group of Hospitals, who is responsible for procuring machinery, maintained 'in procuring any resources, I liaise with the users. If it is x-ray machines, I will liaise with radiographers on the type. Whether I am able to procure what they really want will depend on the resources at my disposal'. The main problem is one of underfunding of Parirenyatwa since independence and a change of Government priorities in the health sector. The Health Services Administrator at Parirenyatwa Hospital pointed out,

> the situation before independence excluded most people from coming to Parirenyatwa hospital, but now everyone is able to. At the same time, Government has diverted the resources to primary health care, which was previously neglected. The Structural Adjustment Program has brought its own stringent measures which has made things harder for the health sector. There have also been inflationary tendencies, with all the prices going up. The devaluation of the dollar has meant that equipment and other resources that require a foreign currency component are much more expensive and often cannot be procured.

All of the doctors interviewed complained that often they are not able to carry out necessary diagnostic tests because of breakdowns in machinery in the wards and in the pathology and x-ray departments. Indeed, they described most of the machinery as 'obsolete', remarking that basic equipment such as ECG machines are often out of order for long periods of time. At any one point in time some of the diagnostic equipment is not working, making it impossible for physicians to establish the correct diagnosis, meaning that they often commence treatment by a process of trial and error. One SRMO described a common ploy adopted by doctors when

116

they suspect the presence of an infection, but cannot carry out the necessary diagnostic test: 'One ends up just prescribing broad spectrum drugs, hoping that they will somehow treat whatever condition the patient has. More often than not treatment is effective, but at the end of the day a doctor does not know what he or she is dealing with'.

Even the Minister of Health described the state of equipment at Parirenyatwa Hospital in the following way, 'X-ray machines which are frequently inoperative, equipment which has a very little degree of reliability and cannot provide emergency ambulatory services' (*Herald*, 25 September, 1990). At the time that interviews were carried out in May 1994, only one of the five imaging machines in the hospital was in functional order. Consequently, fairly ordinary procedures such as barium meals could not be carried out and under those circumstances only those who could afford to pay for use of private facilities could be accurately diagnosed. According to the Health Services Administrator, one of the main problems is that hospital equipment is procured from different countries, depending on the price and, sometimes, political expediency. Not surprisingly, locally trained hospital equipment technicians are not able to repair the wide variety of machines available in the hospital and the problem is compounded by very high turnover of these technicians due to dissatisfaction with the low salaries at Government institutions. One surgeon commented thus about the state of equipment at the hospital,

> There are no qualified maintainers ... they do more damage than repair ...
> Out of five machines, only one is working. Now patients wait up to one
> week without investigations. Sometimes ops are carried out without
> investigations and this results in unnecessary operations. Operations now
> take longer. Patient care is compromised. (Surgeon)

All of the doctors interviewed complained about long delays in getting simple routine test results from the laboratories so that, by the time the results get back to the ward, the patient has often been discharged. One SHO who did a two-month attachment at a British hospital complained, 'blood tests take days or weeks here when they take a matter of hours elsewhere, an ultra sound booking is three months and a thyroid function test takes two weeks and by that time the patient has left or you have moved to another firm'.

One SRMO pointed out 'in some countries, all the essential tests are carried out on admission but here it takes two to three days. When I was a student you could carry out all the tests that you wanted'. Some of the doctors allege that the degree of accuracy of results from government laboratories is compromised by a heavy reliance on student technicians and technologists. Although laboratory personnel are trained at Parirenyatwa Hospital, most of them leave as soon as they have fulfilled their contractual obligations due to comparatively poor working conditions at Government institutions. Junior doctors were particularly bitter about the delays which they said got them into trouble with their consultants. A senior registrar in the Department of Pathology confirmed the delays and attributed some of them to a

> shortage of materials like films. As a result, sometimes we produce sub-optimal results. We have particular problems with laboratory tests like urine and blood tests. We do not have an audit system to determine the degree of accuracy but the bottom line is that we need new equipment.

Delays and inefficiency in the paramedical departments have partly been attributed to staff shortages and poor morale but apparently the worst time of all was in November, 1993 when all the laboratory technologists and technicians went on strike and physicians could not get any tests done. A senior registrar in the Pathology Department conceded that the persisting disgruntlement due to unaddressed dissatisfaction with working conditions was affecting the quantity and quality of output in the department.

During the period in which the interviews were conducted, the X-ray Department was only able to carry out urgent x-rays because of a shortage of radiographers since, of the forty posts for radiographers, only 26 are filled and, even if all the posts were filled, the department would still be short-staffed, as is evident from Table 2.1, column 2 which gives the ideal number of radiographers necessary for the size of the department. In addition, out of an establishment of three radiologists, only one post is filled and this radiologist serves both Parirenyatwa and Harare Hospitals, a very unsatisfactory situation. Clearly, the autonomy of all levels of doctors at Parirenyatwa to carry out essential diagnostic tests is curtailed by problems emanating from the economic welfare of the patients and that of the institution itself.

Doctors' Autonomy in Prescribing

After identifying an illness, physicians would naturally like to prescribe the most effective drugs available. Based on this logic, I assumed that adoption of the Essential Drugs List of Zimbabwe (EDLIZ) would constrain doctors' autonomy to prescribe the drugs of their choice. An attempt was therefore made to discover the impact of EDLIZ and any other factors on autonomy in prescribing.

The Deputy Director of Pharmaceutical Services in the Ministry of Health and Child Welfare informed me in interview that there was opposition from pharmacists, doctors, private drug manufacturers and retailers alike when the idea of a limited list was first introduced in the mid-1980s, but that this has largely died down. In a personal interview, the president of the Zimbabwe Medical Association explained that ZMA opposed EDLIZ on the grounds that it 'removed the doctor's freedom to prescribe what he [she] wants and what he [she] thinks best'. The government went ahead and established the list in spite of the opposition, although this may have contributed to the wide consultation that took place. But now, all the different parties, which include government officials, all levels of doctors and pharmacists in public institutions, have widely accepted EDLIZ. Most doctors consider it more-or-less as a 'medical bible' which provides them with answers to most of their common medical problems. The President of the College of Primary Care Physicians of Zimbabwe proudly explained, 'we were consulted and we made an input. We think it is very good ... We encourage our members to use EDLIZ'.

All junior doctors explained that they do not find EDLIZ constricting at all. One JRMO summed up the sentiment expressed by all of them, 'very handy! The new one is very comprehensive. At my level, anything that I want to prescribe is there [list]'. None of those interviewed had ever felt the need to prescribe drugs outside EDLIZ. Even registrars did not find EDLIZ constricting. All the consultants interviewed also accepted the rationale behind EDLIZ and none expressed dissatisfaction with the idea of a limited list, which they agreed met most of their needs. One senior consultant expressed this view, 'EDLIZ eliminates the doctors' belief of 'newest equals best and most expensive'. Inappropriate prescribing is eliminated. EDLIZ assists doctors to make correct decisions. I don't feel restricted by EDLIZ'.

However, the consultants did express concern that most of the drugs on EDLIZ are very old and felt that the list ought to include newer drugs.

119

One consultant also complained that even though as consultants they can order drugs outside EDLIZ, whenever they ask the Ministry of Health and Child Welfare for permission to do so, 'you are told there is no money'. All levels of doctors expressed disappointment and frustration that the establishment of an essential drugs list has not helped the drug supply situation at Parirenyatwa Hospital which, they complained, is very erratic. Even antibiotics which are used very heavily in the hospital are often not available, leading to frustration and sometimes desperation, as one junior doctor illustrated,

> at one time there was no anti-diarrhoeal drug at the hospital. That was absolutely awful ... It is very frustrating when you have to hold a patient's hand and tell them that they are suffering from something that is curable but there are no medicines in the hospital.

Another junior doctor explained,

> A lot of drugs are not available. This is very frustrating. Initially, I was diligent but I gave up because I realised that I was wasting my time. I used to run around looking for drugs for patients in the intensive care unit, but now I just ask the relatives to buy.

It was quite evident from the interviews that all levels of doctors are exasperated with the drug supply situation because, as we have seen, they know that with the right drugs most patients can get well. As in the case of diagnostic tests, when the necessary drugs are available in the hospital pharmacy the needs of SDF patients are well met, but the problem arises when they are not available, because the patients have to procure the drugs for themselves and most cannot afford to buy from the more expensive private pharmacies. One registrar summed up sentiments expressed by most doctors about the drug situation 'the problem is that there are shortages of all drugs. The drugs are not available for SDF patients. One has to make use of whatever is available'. The general health insurance schemes to which most people with health insurance subscribe do not include payment for drugs, and as a result, some paying patients cannot afford to buy drugs in private pharmacies.

One medical lecturer in the Department of Community Medicine of the University of Zimbabwe explained that those responsible for ordering drugs generally underestimate the institutions' drug needs by, for example, not ordering more malaria drugs during the rain season when malaria is prevalent, thus resulting in acute seasonal shortages. One consultant complained that the main problem in the Ministry of Health is that those in charge lack management skills, 'if they have the training, they are hiding it … This country is run by people who cannot manage. If they can; they do not want to'. The World Bank (1992) pointed out that drug shortages were due to both poor management and underfunding.

In spite of the fact that EDLIZ has been described as 'brilliant' by junior doctors and 'quite successful' by government officials, its establishment has led to some loss of autonomy in that doctors cannot choose what they want and think is most effective. But, ultimately, loss of autonomy derives principally from shortage of drugs in the pharmacy at Parirenyatwa. Taking into account the financial realities of the country, it is evident that the drug supply situation would not have been better without EDLIZ and in fact, from, 1981 to the time of adoption of EDLIZ was progressively becoming worse. In, 1983, medical practitioners and pharmacists warned,

> … shortages will get rapidly worse soon unless Government acts to relieve the 'serious' position. Certain types of antibiotics, important diuretics, and preparations used to treat hypertension, asthma, eye ailments and other medications including anti-depressants are in very short supply now. (*Financial Gazette*, 25 February, 1983)

I contend that there has been little loss of autonomy to prescribe arising from the limited list since it has grown progressively comprehensive with each revision and consultants' need for more complex drugs has been catered for within the list. Moreover, doctors from all sectors of the health sector were consulted on the drawing of the list as is clear from examining the list of participants attending the various workshops organised by the Ministry of Health to consult and sensitise health workers.

Without EDLIZ, doctors would probably go for the latest and relatively more expensive drugs, thus reducing the total supply of drugs that can be bought with the limited amount of money allocated to the Parirenyatwa Group of Hospitals. Access to a wide range of drugs would not enable the Ministry of Health to take advantage of the economies of scale in ordering possible with EDLIZ; the money allocated for drugs would not go very far. Thus, rather than the Government policy of EDLIZ reducing doctors autonomy in a rational and systematic way, doctors as a collective would deprive each other of the autonomy to prescribe. A World

Bank report noted that there is a lot of wastage from over-prescribing (World Bank, 1992), an observation confirmed by the Medical Superintendent of the Parirenyatwa Group of Hospitals who stated, 'there is a lot of wastage ... Right now there is an overall syndrome whereby doctors prescribe more drugs than are necessary'. The World Bank's (1992) recommendation that the number of drugs which a doctor prescribes for an outpatient should be limited to two or three drugs has not been systematically enforced by either the Ministry of Health or the Parirenyatwa Hospital administration.

Doctors' Autonomy in Treatment

An assessment of doctors' autonomy in treatment indicates that this is compromised by a shortage of medical and paramedical staff, overwork, shortage or breakdown of equipment and other resources; the economic status of the patient and the doctors' desire to meet their own economic needs.

In a teaching hospital, one of the principal roles of consultants and heads of medical firms is to teach and supervise those under them in the hierarchical firm structure (see Figure 5.1 below). Each medical firm is supposed to comprise a consultant who is also head of the firm; a senior registrar; government medical officers; senior house officers; junior and senior resident medical officers. Some firms do not have senior registrars because this is the category of doctors which has left the country in large numbers while others have expatriate registrars. A typical firm structure is illustrated in Figure 5.1.

The hospital has a shortage of all grades of doctors, but the situation is worse for registrars, with only twelve of the twenty six posts in the hospital filled (MOH, 1994). The problem is compounded by the fact that a number of doctors of all ranks occupy shared posts and work at both Parirenyatwa and Harare hospitals. The Ministry of Health explains that it has failed to monitor and control the movements of these doctors who often claim that they are at one hospital when they are at neither and may, in fact, be doing private work (Comptroller and Auditor General, 1995).

Figure 5.1   The Medical Firm Structure

Medical Superintendent

↑

Consultant

↑

Senior Registrar

↑

Junior registrar/General Medical
Officer/Senior House Officer

↑

Junior/ Senior Resident Medical Officer

The junior doctors complained that in addition to the shortage of medical staff, they look after too many patients, making their workload excessively heavy as one senior house officer working in an ophthalmology firm explained,

> The workload which we have as doctors prohibits us from practising medicine as we should. We were taught to sit down with a patient and examine them carefully and explain the procedure including the side effects. I find I am not able to do any of that because I am far too busy. I have hundreds of patients waiting to be seen and, as a result, I tend to disregard their general condition and only focus on the eyes.

A registrar in the same department who has also worked in two other African countries concurred with his junior's sentiments,

> I see between 100 to 150 patients a day. There are far too many patients and not enough doctors, which means that doctors here work much harder than anywhere else. This reduces the time that an individual doctor spends with a patient.

A senior consultant also complained that in his firm he had no registrar and found himself doing 'trivial work' which should have been done by junior doctors which left him little time to teach and supervise his subordinates.

One of the consequences of medical staff shortage and the ensuing excess workload is that junior doctors at Parirenyatwa find themselves doing

123

most of the work, some of it well above their level of experience, without supervision. In interviews, junior doctors alleged that most consultants do not do their share of work because they spend more time in their private offices when they should be at Parirenyatwa Hospital leaving the juniors overworked and unable to practise medicine effectively. One JRMO complained,

> As housemen we do most of the work. We are almost independent. A consultant see new patients and problem ones. This should be every morning, but this is not always the case. If there is a registrar who is senior, the consultant leaves him to do all the work and the consultant rarely comes. If as a houseman they feel that you know most of the procedures, they leave the ward to you. Most seniors say that you are only supposed to watch a procedure once and then you perform it. In developed countries and some African countries, consultants do less medical and surgical work than Zimbabwean junior doctors. Here consultants teach you everything in the first week so that you know, but primarily so that they can go away and leave you to do everything.

Most junior doctors complained that they learnt how to perform medical/surgical procedures from peers of the same grade and the one commonly cited procedure in this regard is the Caesarean section. One SRMO explained, 'I watched one, did one with assistance and thereafter I am doing them on my own ... I am more experienced now'. Another SRMO alleged that, 'we are rarely taught by a consultant. They are mostly not there so they cannot teach a junior'. A senior resident medical officer argued, 'The problem is that once some superiors know that you can do certain procedures, they never want to do the procedure themselves, but you also want to learn from the senior. Some consultants even fail you or give you a bad report so that you repeat that stage and continue to do the work while they do their own private work.

All junior doctors stated that it is not unusual for them to admit, carry out diagnostic tests, treat and discharge a patient who has not ever been seen by a consultant. They maintained that the amount of supervision by seniors varies from firm to firm, but all agreed that it is below standard, with the Obstetrics and Gynaecology Department which is the busiest in the hospital, being the most 'notorious' for lack of supervision. These sentiments were confirmed by some registrars, consultants, Ministry of Health senior officials and the Comptroller and Auditor General, who investigated the provision of health services and personnel utilisation at

Zimbabwe's central and provincial hospitals in 1995. It would seem that the problems experienced in Zimbabwe are not unique, since Yates (1995) has also found that some NHS consultants treat their private patients when they should be working on NHS patients, giving rise to long waiting lists in departments where such practises are common.

Most junior doctors complained that they frequently do the ward rounds on their own, as one SRMO explained, 'here I often do rounds on my own. I provide minimum care especially when dumped in the Casualty department alone. This dampens any enthusiasm to learn'. One senior house officer who did a two-month elective period at a British hospital explained that in Zimbabwe he had much less teaching and supervision by his seniors but had a much heavier workload and a lot more experience with patients than his British counterparts. He complained that while the experience was valuable, the junior doctors at Parirenyatwa become over-confident and take risks carrying out operations without adequate experience. The point was often made that expatriate registrars were less experienced than Zimbabwean senior resident medical officers. One junior doctor explained, 'here, SRMOs do serious surgical work like skull operations on their own. You become over-confident and overlook your limits and expose patients to unnecessary risks'. The Medical Superintendent of Parirenyatwa Hospital affirmed that some of the deaths in the hospital are caused by inexperienced junior doctors carrying out delicate and serious operations because the senior doctors are not available (Comptroller and Auditor General, 1995).

A registrar in the Ophthalmology Department who was studying for a Masters degree in Medicine complained that his supervision was less than what it should be, but the department only had one consultant instead of three. Another registrar in the Orthopaedic Department who was in his fourth year of studying for a Masters degree mentioned that he got virtually no supervision from his consultant, who left all the work to him, making it impossible for him to study for his degree programme. He stated that he does most of the procedures on his own but where he is not sure, he is supposed to tell his consultant because if he makes a mistake he gets into trouble. In interview, the Minister of Health complained, 'paying for ghost doctors cannot be a good environment for the young doctors'. In another context he confirmed that government and university-employed consultants were devoting more time to private patients at the expense of Government patients (*Herald*, 29 May, 1994) and that there is no mechanism for monitoring the time they spent in the hospital.

All grades of doctors complained that the shortage of all categories of support workers, but especially nurses, had seriously compromised general patient care as one SRMO points out, 'doctors do not work in isolation. Shortage of staff compromises treatment and monitoring. For example, hourly blood pressure checks are necessary sometimes, but often in the ward there is only a nurse and a student nurse and they cannot carry out all the checks that you want'. A surgeon summed up the situation as follows,

> there is a shortage of all grades of health workers. There is need for more nurses who are the back bone of the health services in Zimbabwe. Basic nursing care is no longer given. As a result there is little support for doctors. I often ask myself whether a patient will survive on the ward after surgery.

The Deputy Minister of Health claimed that the shortage of nurses and doctors in government hospitals had become 'desperate and critical' and she recommended that the hospitals should be declared a 'national disaster' to force the government to act urgently on the problem. She said that more nurses were needed in order to deal with a serious congestion in the wards, partly resulting from the AIDS pandemic (*Sunday Mail*, 2 January 1994). Doctors complained that a shortage of staff in other departments, such as the Physiotherapy Department, meant that doctors were not able to refer patients there for rehabilitation (see Table 2.1). The Medical Superintendent of Parirenyatwa Hospital remarked that the hospital needed 'six speech therapists but it did not have even one' (*Herald*, 11 March 1993).

A shortage of equipment in the wards and theatres has made it difficult for doctors not only to diagnose but also to treat patients effectively. Junior doctors complained that there is a general shortage of gloves, linen, and surgical instruments such as those used in urology and orthopaedic surgeons complained about shortages of prosthetic equipment in their department. One senior surgeon complained that the shortage of equipment is frustrating because one is 'working in an environment which does not allow one to do what you were taught. Surgery needs hi-tech equipment and it is just not available at Parirenyatwa'. He argued that the situation is deteriorating to become like Kenya, 'where five surgeons carry out one operation because of a shortage of surgical equipment'.

Consultants, particularly surgeons, complained about the lack of more recent equipment which would enable them to carry out the latest techniques and attend to more complicated cases. One surgeon mentioned that some of the Zimbabwean patients going to South Africa for heart operations are being operated on by Zimbabwean doctors working there but if the cardiac equipment at Parirenyatwa were in working order, these operations could be done in Zimbabwe and the foreign currency currently being paid to South African hospitals would benefit more Zimbabweans. In fact, open heart surgery was carried out at Parirenyatwa by a medical team from Loma Linda University in California in 1988 and it was expected that a local team of cardiologists whom they worked with, would continue, but this did not happen (*Sunday Mail*, 12 February,1989). Instead, the Cardiac Unit was closed down in 1990 due to lack of purfussionists to operate the lung machine and, in addition, Z$2 million worth of new equipment such as artificial valves was needed to make the machine functional.

The state of the equipment in the hospital is not surprising, given that most of it was bought in 1974 when the main complex was commissioned and, since then, replacement has been piecemeal (MOH & CW Committee Report, 1994). The deplorable state of most of the equipment at Parirenyatwa was described by the Parliamentary Committee looking at service ministries in 1993, 'Your committee was shown lots of obsolete equipment in the various Intensive Care units, the Electronic and Mechanical departments, the Central Sterilising Supplies Department (CSSD) and X-ray Department' (Parliament of Zimbabwe Vote No.15-1990-1991). These findings were confirmed by a technical committee set up to assess the functioning of the hospital in 1994 (MOH & CW, 1994). The state of medical equipment at Parirenyatwa has meant that doctors of all grades are unable to effectively diagnose and treat patients.

According to the journal *Africa Health*, the shortage and breakdown of hospital equipment is common in most African countries. The journal predicted, 'sixty per cent of the new medical equipment (in cost terms) which is bought, loaned or given to Africa will not be working by next year and by 1992, twenty per cent more will not be working' (cited in *Herald*, 8 November, 1990).

Assessing the Influence of Some Principal Factors on Clinical Autonomy

Peer Review through the Firm Structure

A system of peer review serves to identify and correct dangerous practices in patient care, identify procedures and practices which are unnecessarily expensive, and to provide data on doctors' own practises which can improve their efficiency (Freddi, 1989). The medical firm structure is a type of peer review with in-built checks and balances by which clinical decisions made by junior doctors are reviewed by their seniors. At the same time, the presence of juniors is supposed to make seniors, who serve as both teachers and role models, more conscientious and vigilant in their clinical performance. As discussed earlier, this structure is not working efficiently at Parirenyatwa and the decisions made by junior doctors are often final because the senior doctors do not regularly have rounds and undertake other medical duties with their juniors. Under those circumstances, junior doctors exercise more autonomy than would be the case if the medical firm structure was working.

Medical/Surgical Audit

The recently introduced audit system is another factor which might, on the face of it, reduce medical autonomy, but on closer inspection, however, it has a minimal impact for a number of reasons. The idea of audit was first suggested by the President of the Zimbabwe Medical Association in 1992 in the wake of public moral outrage following allegations of malpractice levelled at one private anaesthetist, Dr McGowan (discussed in detail in Chapter 7). After the release of a report of the Parliamentary Select Committee appointed to look at the functions of the Health Professions Council, the President of the ZMA announced that the medical profession was going to adopt medical audit to police itself (*Herald*, 4 March, 1993).

The objective of adopting the audit system, as announced publicly, is that of policing medical practice and safeguarding the welfare of the patients, but the hidden agenda is that of forestalling the imposition of a Government-sponsored audit scheme which is likely to be more stringent. As one senior registrar pointed out, 'the issue of surgical audit should be taken seriously. We should do it ourselves, before the politicians get involved. Politicians are asking a lot of questions on how misconduct is dealt with'. This reaction is very similar to that of the British medical profession which delayed the adoption of medical audit for a long time and when it was made mandatory in 1989, doctors opted for managerial positions in the NHS in order to ensure that would not implemented by non-medical management (Dent, 1995; Hunter, 1994).

However, surgical audit is in place in some departments at Parirenyatwa but not in others. In fact, the term is currently used to describe a variety of events and most doctors are not clear about how the present audit system works, largely because of its variations in different departments. Surgical, paediatric, anaesthetic, and obstetric and gynaecology departments have adopted audit systems of some sort. In some of the departments, audit is referred to as mortality meetings which are held at intervals ranging from monthly up to every six months while in others, the ward clerk simply collates statistics on admissions, deaths and discharges. One surgeon stated that he has monthly audit lunch meetings with all members in his firm, including the nurses, and they discuss the outcomes of all neurosurgical cases operated on by his firm during the previous month. While this is commendable, there is no-one to comment on his own performance and this applies to all departments where there is only one consultant in the whole specialty.

In the departments which have adopted audit, all the doctors of the specialty or department meet to review complicated cases, deaths and any unusual or interesting cases which have occurred. The presenter discusses the presenting symptoms; the diagnostic tests carried out; findings; treatment, including surgery; and the patient outcome and colleagues comment, criticise and advise on what could have been done, if they have a different view.

Everyone in the firms that have audit systems said they are supposed to attend the meetings although they do not always do so, but unfortunately, there is no mechanism for enforcing attendance because audit was spearheaded by the ZMA and not by Government or the Parirenyatwa Hospital management. How seriously audits are taken varies from firm to firm but junior doctors normally attend because of their involvement in the day-to-day management of patients, although most dislike the meetings which they refer to as 'witch hunting' because they think that the idea is to find out who is to blame for deaths and other fatal mistakes. Some argued that exposure of one's mistakes before colleagues made one feel incompetent while those who were in favour of the audit system stated that the meetings provided constructive criticism.

Registrars and consultants in firms with audit systems emphasized that the aim of audit systems was for medical practitioners to correct and learn from each other not witch hunting. In these terms, one senior surgeon argued that 'the public think it is there to find out who did what but, in fact, audit is meant to improve the quality of service and to get others' opinions'.

It appears that the doctors at Parirenyatwa are, like their British counterparts, in favour of audit which focuses on the process rather than outcome of care (Hunter, 1994).

The conclusion from an assessment of the audit system as it exists at present at Parirenyatwa is that it is largely ineffective in influencing doctors' clinical practices, the main reason being that the scheme was introduced by doctors and not by the Government and there are no sanctions in place. It is highly unlikely that doctors would introduce a system which results in loss of their clinical autonomy. Audit has been introduced to deflect public attention from the medical profession, to limit the damage done to the profession's public image by the publicity following the McGowan case and evidently, to arrest any efforts by the Government to introduce a more effective audit system.

The effectiveness of the system in monitoring doctors' behaviour is reduced by the fact that not all cases handled by firms are discussed since doctors choose the cases that they want to present, leaving the possibility that firms may not bring out cases that were really disastrous because they do not want to show their gross mistakes to colleagues. In addition, the varying intervals between audits within individual departments can mean that the impact of the criticism is often lost because the junior doctors and registrars involved may have moved to other departments.

Despite the caveats, the voluntary introduction of the system by doctors, regardless of the objective and its effectiveness, indicates that there has been some shift in the power of the medical profession. Previously, their practice behaviour was never questioned, but now the profession is on the defensive.

Cost Containment

In the face of such wide ranging problems due to financial constraints experienced by the hospital and the Government as a whole, one would expect that some stringent and systematic cost containment measures would have been taken by the institution or the Ministry of Health to alter the nature of individual doctors' diagnosis and therapy patterns since these account for 80 per cent of health costs in a hospital (Dohler, 1989), but this has not happened. In the United States and Britain, specific mechanisms aimed at cost reduction, such as diagnosis related groups, clinical protocols and secondary surgical opinion have been adopted (Dent, 1995; Dohler, 1989). In the Zimbabwean context, the overall budget for health care has been reduced since the introduction of ESAP, as pointed out in Chapter 4, and patients are responsible for most of their health care costs, but the physicians have retained their clinical autonomy within the limits imposed by the budget, as happened in Britain before the introduction of the NHS reforms in the late 1980s (Klein, 1989). A junior doctor decides on a course of action and, more often than not, carries it out without a second opinion from his or her senior to confirm its efficacy and cost effectiveness. The lack of systematic cost control mechanisms, however, means that doctors' autonomy is also restricted by the wastefulness of other doctors (Light, 1995). But doctors have been compelled to alter their clinical behaviour as a result of the financial difficulties facing some of their patients, the hospital and the Government as a whole. However, in the absence of systematic and effective cost containment measures, the extent to which doctor's clinical behaviour has been affected varies widely.

As mentioned earlier, doctors do not pay much attention to cost when dealing with non-paying SDF patients, simply, what they are able to do for them depends on what is available at that time. All of those interviewed stated that they are cost conscious when attending to paying patients, including those on medical aid who may have to pay for shortfall out of their pocket if the bill is too high. Doctors nostalgically looked back to the period prior to the rationalisation of hospital fees when clinical decisions were only determined by the physical condition of the patient and the availability of resources. They explained that since then some paying patients ask to be released before they are fit in order to reduce their hospital bill. One SRMO described one of his experiences as follows,

> Since the introduction of hospital fees, I have tried to reduce the drugs that I prescribe and the number of days that a patient has to stay in hospital. I may discharge a patient before they are fully recovered in order to reduce the cost. One time I discharged a patient four days after a major operation. The abdominal wound was healing and she was passing water alright and the patient wanted to go home because of the cost. I gave the patient a prescription and about two weeks later, the patient came back in a worse condition than before the operation since she had not bought the prescribed drugs, as she did not have any money. She died a day after readmission, which was very frustrating for me.

In fact, the level of cost consciousness in the treatment of non-paying patients varies widely with some doctors claiming that they are cost conscious because they feel that resources will go further. As one registrar stated, 'you use one pair of gloves where two would have been better because of AIDS, but you think of the cost'. Another registrar in the Ophthalmology Department pointed out that he always used to carry out diagnostic tests before surgery but that he no longer does, unless he thinks that it will significantly help the patient. He said that previously if a patient's operation was cancelled for administrative reasons, they would stay in hospital, but now they have to go home and come back on the scheduled day, which is a change from past practice. Most doctors pointed out that in cases where there are obvious HIV symptoms, they tend to be more cost conscious as one SRMO explained,

> If I have two patients, one who is HIV positive and another who is negative, I tend to be more aggressive with the negative one because he is likely to be productive and help us to procure drugs in future. If it were not for the cost I would treat them equally, but now if I give someone who is positive expensive drugs I will deprive someone who is likely to have a longer life.

The existence of AIDS-related symptoms gives doctors the autonomy to decide whether or not to use scarce resources on patients likely to die in the near future. What is disturbing is the fact that the decision is based on suspicion, rather than HIV testing, which is only supposed to be carried out when necessary, because of the costs of HIV tests, the need to respect a patient's privacy and protection from prejudice because of their illness. Ironically, this does not seem to give patients any protection and, in fact, it is likely that a few patients who are not HIV positive may find themselves denied adequate treatment because their illness appears consistent with HIV symptoms. Treatment of HIV patients gives doctors working in the medical wards more autonomy in that they have not introduced medical audits allegedly because a large number of the patients in those wards have AIDS-related illnesses. AIDS is now the biggest killer in the 25-44 age group in Zimbabwe, accounting for 25 per cent of the deaths and 14.2 per cent of all deaths in the country and taking up 27 per cent of all health care expenditure (*Parade*, July 1996:6). Thus, where doctors in other disciplines are introducing mechanisms to make each other more accountable, those in medical wards are becoming more relaxed in this respect because most of their patients are assumed to be terminal cases.

One surgeon asserted,

> I am very cost conscious. If I want government to pay me more, I must not waste resources. Efficiency does not co-habit with waste. Custodians of resources in health services are doctors. We prescribe, we need to be cost conscious. I am renowned for my attitude towards waste. If a nurse opens a suture that I am not going to use, I tell her off.

One senior registrar said that he is cost conscious, 'to an extent, but probably not as much as I should be' and this sums up the attitude of most of the doctors interviewed. One senior consultant commented,

> Yes, we have to reduce costs. Audit helps because we ask why a doctor is keeping a patient too long. He or she must give appropriate treatment. Costs cannot be regulated in medicine. Those who want to control medicine fail here. The same op can take one hour by one person and three hours by another.

The above surgeon's remarks show that he is not in favour of cost-containment measures introduced by management but prefers those from colleagues through the audit process which, as we saw earlier, is too infrequent and optional. A few doctors mentioned that they were deliberately not cost conscious when dealing with non-paying patients on whom they would rather use resources 'than have the money go to Ministers' fuel or allowances'.

Doctors' Financial Needs

Doctors' preoccupation with their own economic needs has compromised clinical performance as senior doctors carry out private work during working hours leaving junior doctors to do most of the work. Juniors are also doing locum work, often during working hours and both claim that their economic needs are so inadequately met by their government remuneration that they have to create the time for private work. All the doctors argue that the government should provide them with a 'living wage' to enable them to practise medicine in the best possible way.

The Ministry of Health and Child Welfare officials admit that private work, particularly that carried out during working hours, is seriously compromising clinical practice at Parirenyatwa and other government institutions. One junior doctor stated, the Z$2000 [approximately 200 pounds sterling] that I clear at the end of the month is inadequate for my needs and, as a result, most of us have to put in extra hours somewhere else during working hours. This is unfortunate because this means that one does not put all their effort in the government hospital but steals a few hours during working hours and explains it somehow.

Some explicitly said that they do the minimum possible in the government hospital in order to create time for locum work. One SRMO recognised that patients may suffer as a result of private work, but still felt that 'self preservation and self survival is the first principle of nature. We have to live'. In the same vein, a senior registrar argued that, 'total patient care is no longer there for both junior and senior doctors because you will starve. Patient care has therefore been compromised'.

Clearly, medical practice in Zimbabwean government hospitals is underpinned by the economic situation of the government and its institutions, the carers and the patients themselves. Doctors are not only leaving patients in hospital to attend to private patients in their private rooms, but government and university-employed consultants are allegedly devoting more time to their private patients within government hospitals at the expense of public patients (*Herald*, 29 May, 1994).

Statutory Instrument 93 of 1993

In 1993, the Government of Zimbabwe passed Statutory Instrument 93 of the Medical Dental and Allied Professions Act (Chapter 224) with the intention of forcing medical practitioners to report on each others' behaviour. This was passed in response to allegations against anaesthetist Dr McGowan, who carried out more than 500 experiments on unsuspecting patients, some of whom died while others were disabled, from 1985 to 1990 (*Herald*, 4 March, 1993). The public was angry that none of the surgeons and nurses who worked with him reported anything, even though most of them were unhappy with what was happening. According to Instrument 93, any health worker who commits, participates or witnesses improper or disgraceful conduct, gross incompetence or malpractice by a health worker or institution is legally bound to report to the Health Professions Council within fourteen days, or they too will be liable for prosecution.

I assumed that this regulation would erode clinical autonomy by making medical practitioners more cautious in their work for fear of being reported. However, all of the junior doctors interviewed, except two, stated that they were not aware of the regulation. After I had explained the terms of the Instrument, all those interviewed, except one, stated that they would not report a medical colleague and one JRMO categorically stated, 'I would never report a colleague as stipulated in that regulation. That will create enemies and ruin someone's career'. Yet another JRMO pointed out,

> I would discuss it with them nicely, rather than reporting. We don't do that. If there is a report to be made it has to come from the patient. Sisters can report. They have that kind of power. Sisters can report to the consultant. We have not been told to report each other.

In similar terms, one SHO described her experience as follows: 'no I would not report a colleague. One time, my colleague who was the anaesthetist was drunk in theatre and the sister in theatre phoned the consultant and he was sent home'. The above comments confirm Freidson's (1988) observation that physicians give each other the benefit of the doubt to the extent not done in other occupations. Rosenthal (1995) found the same unwillingness to report on colleagues by doctors in Britain, Sweden and the United States and attributes this to the level of uncertainty in much of medical work.

One SRMO who is an official of HDA, declared that he would not follow the regulation since, in his opinion, the problem was one of failure to act by government and its officials who know what is happening but do not want to act on it. He gave an example of illegal abortions by doctors arguing,

> the number of abortions in this country is so high, they are a way of family planning. If government does not want to do something about it why should I waste my time? Medicine is a very closed profession. We support each other. You have to have another doctor to convict in a case of malpractice and this is why McGowan's court case [referred to earlier] is not going anywhere.

The President of the ZMA maintained that his organisation did not accept the Instrument, arguing that the reason was that it was passed without consultation, was punitive and doctors would not comply. He declared,

> We are vehemently opposed to that Instrument which was passed in Parliament without consultation of the Health Professions Council or the

Zimbabwe Medical Association. We are greatly opposed to it because of problems of relations with colleagues and, in fact, all health professionals have dismissed it and will not abide by it. There is a great ethical problem of reporting a colleague and this has never happened before. The Instrument does not give room for counselling. It is a bogus law. I do not know anyone who has reported a colleague. We criticise it because it is a statutory instrument and should not be compulsory. It results in bad blood. It punishes one for keeping quiet ... violates human rights.

Concern with the maintenance of good relations with colleagues appears to be central to doctors' unwillingness to 'tell on each other'. Doctors interviewed by Rosenthal (1995) in Britain, Sweden and the United States stated that they would only report if they had a bad relationship with the colleague in question. The regulation is similar to the informer laws which were passed in the United States and which have been effective in breaking medical silence and forcing doctors to testify against each other in a court of law (Freidson, 1989). From the comments, it is quite clear that Instrument 93 is not likely to be effective in reducing doctors' autonomy, partly because most of the doctors are not aware of its existence, but principally because they are simply not prepared to report each other and risk making enemies and ruining another doctor's career. The regulation can only be as effective as the willingness of the people who apply it but in fact, even other health workers, particularly nurses, are reluctant to report on doctors because they feel that nothing will be done and they just end up souring relations in their work environment for no benefit.

Litigation

A doctor is sued for malpractice when it is suspected that he or she caused injury by not exercising reasonable care customary to standards of the profession (Dingwall, 1994; Feltoe and Nyapadi, 1989). In the United States, there is evidence that doctors faced with the possibility of litigation are likely to be more conscientious in their clinical practices (Harrison and Schulz, 1989). The risk of payment of compensation is supposed to be an incentive for doctors to perform their duties more carefully and limit the possibility of harm to their patients (Dingwall, 1994). In this situation, the doctor's clinical practices may no longer be directed by their professional knowledge alone, but by external constraints, i.e. fear of litigation and payment of compensation. For example, they may carry out more diagnostic tests than they would normally do in order to be absolutely sure of the diagnosis. While this may represent some loss of clinical autonomy, it also increases the income of the physician at the expense of the patient who has to meet higher health costs, as is happening in the United States (Light, 1995).

All the doctors interviewed claimed that fear of litigation does not affect their clinical practices at Parirenyatwa, the main reason being that Zimbabwean patients treated in Government hospitals do not sue their doctors. Junior doctors explained that they do not worry about the possibility of litigation because they are not responsible for the patients that they treat, patients belong to the consultant, and he/she is responsible for the junior doctor's work. One SRMO referred to himself as 'just a hand', without responsibility for the patient.

The fact that doctors themselves do not pay compensation out of their own pocket, even if they were successfully sued, removes any constraints that litigation could have on their clinical behaviour. One doctor summed up the sentiments expressed by many, 'doctors working in government are well protected. It is the responsibility of the senior and at the end of the day, it is the Minister of Health who is sued and government pays the costs'.

All the doctors argued that the conditions under which they work are not ideal and it is to be expected that some mistakes will be made. They pointed to the amount of work that they do and the shortages and other constraints that they work with, explaining that the context of medical practice at Parirenyatwa makes mistakes inevitable. Ironically, they also pointed out that the imperfect medical environment in which they work protects them because it is difficult to establish the cause of injury or death. One registrar explained that there are so many constraints in diagnosing, prescribing and treatment that anything could go wrong, unlike in a private hospital where everything is available. One SRMO declared,

> I cannot be sued in a government hospital. I have no patient therefore if I make a mistake, the people above me are responsible. Government-employed doctors are working under difficult conditions, doing an operation on my own, if I make a mistake people will understand.

All doctors, including the consultants, argued that the patients that they treat in Government hospitals are not aware of their rights and they rarely ever sue the doctor. All junior doctors indicated that they do not know of anyone who has been sued by a patient at Parirenyatwa or any government hospital. One doctor remarked, 'Shona patients are stupid because they keep quite even when things are terrible'. He gave the example of patients 'queuing for hours for treatment without complaining. That is why no one thinks patients will sue them'.

A senior registrar said that he was much more cavalier in his clinical behaviour compared to the US where he did his post-graduate training. He stated that in the US one has to cover all possibilities because the patients sue very easily. One surgeon doubted that anyone would sue because, 'patients here are very stupid. They will grumble, but they will never stand up for themselves. Even when I advise my patients to sue me they will not.' In fact, this characteristic is not confined to Zimbabwean patients only since, as Klein (1987) points out, the propensity to sue is not equally distributed in any society. Evidence from Britain shows that even there most patients do not sue, and when they do, most just want an apology rather than a financial settlement (Dingwall and Fenn, 1992; Rosenthal, 1995).

All doctors mentioned that they also did not expect litigation because of the patients' financial circumstances. One doctor summed up the situation as follows, 'in Zimbabwe it is not a major problem because many of the patients are not aware of their rights. Even if they were, they do not have money for legal costs and the hassles inhibit patients from taking further action'. However, the doctors claimed that they were always careful and aware of the possibility of litigation when dealing with private patients when they are on locum work. One SHO confirmed,

> I am aware of the possibility of litigation with my private patients. I feel more responsible for the patient. The patient is mine and I am dealing with an educated patient. I take lots of precautions to avoid mistakes and negligence. I always ask patients whether they are allergic to certain drugs or not.

In summary, there is little loss of clinical autonomy due to the threat of litigation and the doctors themselves admit that they are not as careful with government patients as they are with private ones because of the constraints under which they work and because of the patients' financial and social position and cultural beliefs. However, some patients and relatives do complain to either hospital management or the Ministry of Health and Child Welfare but, until 1995 when the department of Public Relations was established at Parirenyatwa Hospital, some of the letters of complaint were lost while those that went to the right place were handled in a less than systematic way and, in fact, only those that went as far as litigation were taken seriously.

Culturally, most Zimbabweans believe that misfortunes have their origins in family relationships, particularly with ancestral spirits (Bourdillon, 1982; Chavunduka, 1978). Hence, the cause of death could be attributed to ancestral spirits, which relinquish their protection of the family when displeased, or to bad spirits (Chavunduka, 1978). Under those circumstances, the doctor is only an instrument of imminent death, but he or she is not really responsible because the victim was going to die anyway. In this context, efforts by the family will be devoted to identifying the displeased ancestral spirit and to atonement and propitiation for the mistake. In any case, suing the doctor or whoever is responsible will not bring back the dead person and, as a result, even in cases where negligence is obvious, suing is not considered an option by the majority; the notion that one can benefit from death is foreign to most Zimbabweans.

As has been pointed out by doctors, most patients are not in a financial position to sue a doctor who has the whole Government to defend him or her. The informational distance between the doctor and the patient makes it difficult for patients to say that someone died of anything other than what the doctor has stated, primarily because most people do not have access to medical information and cannot tell when there has been an adverse outcome. The attitudes of most Zimbabweans contradicts Haug's vision of assertive consumers in Western countries who seek to participate in their treatment and are litigious (Haug, 1988). To make matters worse, a suing patient is unlikely to get a doctor to testify as an expert witness because the population of doctors is very small and they all know each other. Their reactions to the possibility of implementing Statutory Instrument 93 of 1993 gives an indication of some of the problems confronting the legal system in the country when it comes to cases concerning medical negligence and malpractice.

Finally, most Zimbabwean patients are genuinely unaware of the options available to them, since most will never have heard of a patient suing a doctor until the McGowan case in 1992. Although the Consumer Council of Zimbabwe drafted a Patients' Rights Charter, its Executive Director admitted that its activities in the health sector are restricted to queries on wrong prescriptions or widely varying prices of drugs in private pharmacies and those with complaints of a clinical nature are referred to the Health Professions Council.

Conclusions

The doctors at Parirenyatwa Hospital have considerable clinical autonomy as a result of minimal regulation by the Ministry of Health, hospital management, and the patients. Unlike their counterparts in the United States and increasingly in Britain, they do not have to contend with clinical guidelines aimed at controlling the quality and cost of health care. Their autonomy is, however, seriously constrained by the general shortage of resources in the hospital and the economic capacity of some of their patients. Thus, although doctors have autonomy in deciding on the type and number of diagnostic tests that they want, their ability to implement these decisions is seriously constrained by the unavailability of essential equipment and the breakdown of that which is available, as well as by the inability of some patients to afford some of the diagnostic tests.

Doctors' autonomy in prescribing has been constrained more by the general shortage of drugs in the hospital and the inability of some patients to procure drugs from private pharmacies than by the existence of EDLIZ, which includes most drugs which the doctors would want to use, although most of them are old. The major constraint which the doctors experience, arises from the general shortage of drugs, which could easily have been worse in the absence of EDLIZ, but since the introduction of ESAP, any constraints that there may have been from EDLIZ no longer apply when dealing with paying patients.

In the treatment and general management of patients, doctors have minimal constraints from administrative regulations, but what they are able to do is determined by the availability of essential resources, support personnel and the economic position of the patient. Shortage of support personnel, such as nurses and physiotherapists, prohibits doctors from prescribing essential observations and rehabilitative procedures. Overwork and all the other constraints have, in fact, released doctors from closer scrutiny, which could have reduced their autonomy in clinical practice. As it is, all levels of doctors are largely left to do what they can with the resources and personnel available, and some have taken advantage of the situation and relaxed because they do not expect to be disciplined under the circumstances.

Doctors do not rigorously account for their clinical behaviour, partly because the firm structure, which is supposed to provide some peer review, is not working efficiently and has been distorted by the shortage of all grades of doctors, particularly that of registrars. This has left junior doctors with much more autonomy and responsibility than they should have for that stage in their careers and this has absolved them from professional accountability for their clinical activities. As for the senior doctors, they cannot possibly carry out all the work that arises as a result of the shortages and society and administrators are expected to understand their plight. This is irrespective of the fact that they are spending a lot of their time doing private work.

Hospital management at the Parirenyatwa Group of Hospitals, as in all other government hospitals, is there to facilitate medical work rather than to control it, to use Harrison and Shulz's (1988) expression. Unlike in the United States and increasingly in Britain, the hospital management at Parirenyatwa is largely advisory rather than directive and prescriptive. Even though the hospital has serious fiscal problems as a result of general under-funding by the Government, little attempt has been made to systematically and significantly reduce the magnitude of expenditure incurred by individual doctors' clinical practices. The constraints on clinical autonomy are less stringent than in the United States, although the shortage of resources is much more severe than in both Britain and the United States.

Instrument 93, which could have gone some way in making doctors more conscientious in their work and protecting the patients at the same time, has not worked as expected because of the unwillingness of the doctors to report on each other. The other potentials weapons which patients could use on their own to protect themselves or redress some wrong doing, which include complaining and litigation, have not been effective to date in the Zimbabwean context, primarily because most are also not in a position to understand the intricacies of medical practice to be able to challenge decisions by a doctor. Even when they do, most patients are not familiar with the channels for complaining and most of them do not have financial resources to initiate litigation. Suing a doctor working at Parirenyatwa means taking on the whole Government, as it were, and, understandably, most find this an intimidating prospect. Finally, patients' cultural beliefs also reduce the possibility of litigation, as explanations for ill-health and death are sought in the spirit world, with doctors being seen merely as the unwitting instruments of spirits.

6 Economic Autonomy

Introduction

This chapter aims to answer the question: to what extent are the different grades of doctors able to determine their remuneration, hours of work and location of work in and outside government employment? The second aim is to assess the extent to which aspects of Government policy affect their economic autonomy.

One of the ongoing debates in theories of the professions concerns the degree of economic autonomy which doctors employed in bureaucratic institutions are able to exercise (Derber *et al*, 1990; Elston, 1991; Freidson, 1988, 1989a, 1989b; McKinlay and Arches, 1985, 1986; McKinlay and Stoeckle, 1988). Proletarianisation advocates claim that professionals employed in bureaucratic organisations are losing control of various prerogatives which they enjoyed as self-employed professionals, including the right to determine their own remuneration, which is now the responsibility of management (Mckinlay and Arches 1985, 1986; McKinlay and Stoeckle, 1988). However, they point out that British consultants have the opportunity to increase their remuneration through the limited private practice that they are permitted. Some theorists contend that even as employees in bureaucratic organisations, doctors still exercise considerable influence in the determination of their conditions of work (Freidson, 1985; Navarro, 1988) and have much more clout in negotiations with employers than other health workers (Elston, 1991). Derber *et al* (1990) claim that professionals are the new mandarins who have been able to convert their main resource, knowledge, into power, status and privilege, which they wield over semi-professionals and clients.

Johnson (1973) who analyzed the nature of autonomy exercised by professionals in post-colonial states claims that doctors have little economic autonomy because their societies offer little opportunity for private work due to the small size of the middle class which can afford such services. In any case, the system of patronage which operates in these countries makes it difficult for doctors to obtain licenses to practise privately. On the other hand, Gish and Martin (1979), who have also looked at the conditions of doctors in developing countries, suggest that they exercise considerable economic autonomy because of their ability to work internationally. They are able to put pressure on governments with threats of migration to countries with better remuneration, thus forcing governments to award them high salaries which they can ill-afford and which distort the income distribution in the country. Doctors' ability to negotiate for high salaries is facilitated by the fact that some policy-makers are themselves doctors (Gish and Martin, 1979). In addition, their negotiating position is enhanced by the high status which they enjoy in their societies, which is also acknowledged by politicians.

This chapter will analyze the extent to which state employment and control of services affect doctors' economic autonomy in post-independence Zimbabwe. It will examine their terms of employment in government, the extent to which they are able to influence their remuneration for services to government, whether or not their employment status allows them to practise privately, the strategies which they adopt in promoting their economic interests, some of the reasons why they enjoy the level of economic autonomy which they do, and the impact of the introduction of free health care and legalisation of traditional medicine on their economic autonomy.

Terms of Doctors' Employment in Government

The employment contracts of government-employed doctors vary according to their grade. Interns work as full-time government employees with a fixed salary, and are entitled to government accommodation near the teaching hospital where they are serving their internship. They have always been prohibited from practising privately, even outside working hours, because they are still in training and are supposed to work under supervision. The employment contract for middle-level doctors, comprising senior house officers, government medical officers, hospital medical officers and registrars, did not allow practising privately on a part-time basis from independence up to 1992. Before independence, full-time government consultants were allowed to carry out private practise both within the hospital and in their own private rooms but, like their British counterparts, they had to forego a twelfth of their government annual salary and (MOH & CW, 1994:9) these conditions did not change after independence. Heads of institutions, departments, districts and provinces, including medical superintendents, on the other hand are prohibited from private practice even during their spare time.

143

The Government White Paper on health released in 1984 states, 'full-time government and university doctors will be expected to respond to this challenge by devoting any 'spare' working time to meet the needs of the people. Private practice by those full-time employees will be phased out' (MOH, 1984:69). Both interns and middle level doctors appear not to have done any private practice up to the late 1980s but, if they did, it was so insignificant that it was no cause for comment by either government officials or the media.

In 1983, the Minister of Health denounced government employed doctors who practised privately (*Herald*, 28 July, 1983) and warned, 'such people must decide whether to become full-time private practitioners or full-time government-employed doctors. There is no question of working on a part-time basis' (ZIANA, 16 August, 1983). In 1984, the Minister complained 'the junior staff complain about lack of supervision because the senior staff are away on private affairs during working hours ... ' (*Herald*, 10 January, 1984). In spite of the government's stance announced in the 1984 White Paper, and although every Minister for the next five years criticised those who practised privately on a part-time basis, no definitive policy decision was taken on the issue until 1989, and no one was ever disciplined.

In 1986, the Public Service Commission carried out an investigation to determine the number of government-employed doctors practising privately and found that 90 per cent of the full-time government consultants among them, a government minister and a deputy minister, practised privately and possibly during working hours (Public Service Commission Report, 29 April, 1986). One of the central problems in the Zimbabwean context is that consultants do not have a contract with the Ministry of Health but with the Public Service Commission, like any other civil servant. Their contracts, like those of their British counterparts, do not specify their exact duties, the minimum number of hours that they should work or the division of labour between them and their juniors in the firm (see Yates, 1995 for a discussion of the British context).

Doctors' dissatisfaction with their working conditions in government was not apparent until they went on strike in 1988, but judging by the levels of turnover from public institutions and some of the speeches made by the Ministers of Health, they were getting increasingly dissatisfied by the mid-1980s (*Herald*, 17 February, 1992). The turnover rates in 1989 were 8.6 per cent for consultants and 21.5 per cent for GMOs, SHOs, and registrars (MOH & CW, 1991) and in 1991, the Ministry of Health lost 39 per cent

144

of its total number of doctors (MOH & CW Staff Establishment List, 1991). Successive Ministers of Health often denounced the doctors for greedy and selfish behaviour and threatened to introduce bonding regulations for medical graduates, even though this was not actually implemented until 1987.

The lack of militancy in demanding better working conditions by junior doctors could partly be attributed to the ease with which they could leave government service for either post-graduate training abroad or to join the vibrant private medical sector in the country. Up to 1987, medical graduates only had to serve a mandatory one year internship before they could leave government service and go into private practice. Another reason for doctors' silence could be that loud demands for better conditions by a group regarded as relatively better off would have been perceived as selfish, at a time when the political rhetoric denounced capitalism and emphasized socialism and equality. The issue of doctors leaving the public sector for the private sector has always been regarded with hostility by government ministers who denounced those who left as unpatriotic and greedy capitalists who were sabotaging government's objective of creating a socialist society. The first Minister of Health argued that he could understand a white person going into private practice but not a black person, 'I can find no mitigating circumstances preventing me from condemning him ... Such profit-motivated parasites, feeding off the ill-health of the community should under no circumstances be tolerated' (*Herald*, 8 October, 1981).

There was a naive assumption that black Zimbabwean doctors had fewer options, as the then Minister of Health argued, 'Now we are training a larger number of blacks, born and bred in Zimbabwe and who have nowhere to go' (*Herald*, 8 December, 1984). In 1987, one Zimbabwean senator asked Government to review the salaries for medical doctors in order to arrest the turnover, pointing out, 'a lot of qualified doctors are leaving the public sector because they earn about five times more as private practitioners ... They are not leaving for love of money but because they cannot make ends meet, especially considering their role and status in society' (*Herald*, 6 March, 1987). No serious attempt was made to significantly improve the conditions of service for doctors in order to retain them even though it was estimated that the country required 4,000 doctors but only had 1,275 registered with the Health Professions Council (Minister of Health's speech on 13 November, 1988) and government was already employing expatriate doctors.

The disparity in income between private and government-employed doctors and their colleagues in full-time private practice grew considerably in the mid-1980s and it was almost inevitable that doctors would leave government service. Government salaries were affected by the devaluation and depreciation of the Zimbabwe dollar since the mid-1980s and this was followed by a steep rise in the cost of houses, cars and other consumer goods. In the early years of independence, pressure to leave government for economic reasons was not so high because, as some doctors explained, one could buy a second hand car, buy a house in a high income area, pay the dowry for a wife, send young siblings to school and improve the economic position of one's parents on a government salary. From the mid-1980s, a doctor working in the public sector could not afford a car and a house and more recently, cannot even afford the rental for a two bedroom flat and buying the basic furniture which they need after leaving government accommodation on completion of internship. Evidently, working in one or other sector makes a tremendous difference to the life styles of doctors and there is, therefore, enormous pressure to leave government employment. As one government doctor explained to me, 'one has to be a fool or very committed to work in government.'

It has generally been accepted in Zimbabwe that the only way for a black person to improve their economic position is through attainment of a good education because all other avenues for advancement, such as entrepreneurial activity, were closed to them during colonialism. Doctors were among the most educated in the society, enjoying both high status and, prestige and logically they were expected to earn more than most people and have a life style to show for it. The economic situation prevailing from the mid-1980s onwards created a disparity between people's expectations and the economic and social reality. This resulted in a high turnover of government employees from all professional categories (Raftopolous, 1986), not just doctors, particularly in the face of government hostility to part-time private practice by its employees. One consultant asked why doctors have to a have a vocation when everybody else, including the socialist politicians, is allowed to make rational economic decisions. She argued that at least doctors are honourable and willing to work for it, while 'your politicians are stealing left, right and centre and you do not say anything'. One JRMO remarked,

Look, society expects us to have a house and a car. I can't buy a house and I can't buy a car. I have nothing. I feel that sitting in an emergency taxi [private estate cars used as public transport and always over-loaded with some passengers sitting in the boot] with my patients is humiliating. Sometimes when I am about to go and sit in the boot, my patients will tell me to come and sit in the front and they sit in the boot.

From the above it is evident that private practice was increasingly no longer for the ethically weak or the politically uncommitted, but was necessary in order to make ends meet. The economic status of doctors and other employed professionals in Zimbabwe is getting increasingly eroded as the national economy slides downwards but this experience is also evident in Kenya. This also occurred in Nicaragua where many revolutionary doctors went into private practice on a part-time basis at least (Garfield and Williams, 1989). The Nicaraguan Government which had initially intended to phase out private practice allowed it to doctors who had completed two years of national service and by 1989, 90 per cent of the doctors practised privately either on a part-time or full-time basis (Garfield and Williams, 1989). The Zimbabwean Government, on the other hand, sought to contain the loss of doctors from its service by bonding locally trained doctors.

The Bonding Contract

In 1987 the Government passed the Medical, Dental and Allied Professions Act which aimed at limiting the growth of the private health sector by arresting the turnover of junior doctors from government institutions, particularly 'white doctors trained at Zimbabwe's expense leaving the country for South Africa. That is why it (government) is bonding' (*Sunday Mail*, 31 March, 1985). The Act increased the period of medical internship from twelve to twenty four months with effect from the beginning of 1988 and those who were already in their first year of internship had to serve a further 12 months. In addition, the Act made it a legal requirement for all medical graduates to work at a designated health institution (government, mission, local authority, selected mine or army hospitals) for five years after internship. Doctors could not be released for post-graduate education unless they were going to specialize in one of the designated critical specialties such as anaesthetics and psychiatry. Those on bonding could be posted wherever there were vacancies but, according to the then Secretary for Health, they could not avoid serving in small outlying hospitals for a period

147

of time (*Herald*, 6 December, 1988). The government made it quite clear that those who did not fulfil their contractual obligations would not be able to practice medicine in Zimbabwe and this made it difficult for doctors to abscond if they hoped to practice in the country later on in their careers.

The legislation was received with hostility by the junior doctors who were going to be affected, white private practitioners, and some members of parliament. Since independence, almost all white medical graduates left the country for post-graduate education in South Africa soon after graduation, without serving their internship in Zimbabwe. They could serve their internship in that country if they so chose. The hostile political relations that existed between the then minority government in South Africa and most of its neighbours meant that Zimbabwe could not ask that government to close that loophole and, up to 1987, the doctors were able to come back to Zimbabwe a few years later as consultants, and go straight into private practice without ever serving in a Zimbabwean government hospital, while their black peers were still working as GMOs at government institutions and waiting for a government scholarship for post-graduate study outside the country.

The new legislation was going to make it difficult for white doctors to return and go straight into private practice, whether as general practitioners or as consultants, and this would affect the quantity of the white private practitioners, as most younger ones had emigrated while those remaining were getting old. This was of serious concern to both the white doctors and the white community which does not normally consult black doctors and, in fact, the adoption of the Medical Dental and Allied Professions Act of 1987 saw a serious drop in the number of white medical students training in the country. White members of parliament were particularly vocal in their opposition to the bill, asking why Zimbabwean doctors had to do a two-year internship when everywhere else it was one year (*Parliamentary Debates*, 31 March, 1987). One white member of parliament declared:

> ... we have got government interference with the profession that is perfectly capable of looking after itself ... I do not support this Bill. It is interfering with a highly professional occupation and will only cause anomalies and stress ... I think it will handicap the growth of the medical profession. It will discourage people from qualifying as doctors. (*Parliamentary Debates*, 26 March, 1987)

The Registrar of the Health Professions Council stated in interview that the Council was also opposed to bonding because it only applied to doctors and not to other health workers. The then Minister of Health justified the policy on the grounds that in developed countries, doctors practice upwards of ten years in government institutions and gain valuable experience before they go into solo practice. He announced that the Practice Control Committee could refuse issuing an open practising license to inexperienced, unscrupulous and inefficient doctors in order to protect the public. The minister further explained,

> You go to Machipisa Shopping Centre [in a low income residential area] and find about seven surgeries, one at every corner. We think it is not necessary and we think when one goes private, we should be able to control where he goes private. There are other needy areas where he will certainly be granted a practising certificate but we wish to discourage a situation where people [doctors] simply go and congregate at one place. (*Parliamentary Debates*, 26 March, 1987)

The passage of the Medical, Dental and Allied Professions Act of 1987 contributed to the resurrection of the dormant Hospital Doctors Association (HDA), originally formed in 1986 as the Junior Hospital Doctors Association (JHDA) (HDA Executive Minutes, 21 October, 1987). Suddenly confronted with the spectre of seven years of Government employment, interns were forced to focus on the level of their remuneration as they had to live on it for much longer. In November 1988, the HDA demanded a reduction in the period of internship as well as in the period they had to work in government and asked the Minister of Health to make a statement to that effect.

The HDA president argued, 'we want the right to decide our own careers, be it post-graduate work or whatever, without being forced to work seven years before doing so' (*Chronicle*, 11 December, 1988). He questioned why only doctors were bonded when every graduate from the University of Zimbabwe is sponsored by government and yet medical graduates still had to pay back the government education loan like every one else. The HDA president pointed out that doctors earned less than laboratory technicians who work a forty hour week, compared to theirs which was much longer. He demanded that doctors receive overtime pay like radiographers and laboratory technicians and warned that interns would no longer do call duty or attend to patients during tea and lunch breaks but would restrict their service to a forty hour week unless the government paid them.

In response, the Secretary for Health asked all heads of department to watch out for any acts of misconduct by junior doctors and charge the offenders in accordance with the Public Service Misconduct Regulations, or negligence (*Herald*, 11 December, 1988). Incensed by the Secretary's response, junior doctors at the four central hospitals went on strike the very next day. They maintained emergency cover in casualty, maternity and neo-natal units, but army doctors had to be called in to assist senior doctors in running all the central hospitals. The ZMA issued a press statement supporting the junior doctors' demands but not the intended strike action (*Herald*, 13 December, 1988). The Secretary General of the Zimbabwe Congress of Trade Unions (ZCTU) sympathized with the doctors' plight, but expressed his opposition to a shortening of the bonding period because of his disapproval of private medicine. He argued that doctors should be prepared to work in rural areas, but 'if they want to become part of the elite that drive around in a Mercedes Benz and milk the *povo* [ordinary people] through their private practices, then we are poles apart' (*Herald*, 15 December, 1988).

The acting Minister of Health stated that he was not going to talk to the doctors unless they went back to work, but promised to look into their grievances within a week. After handing a comprehensive document outlining their grievances to the Ministry of Health they resumed work after three days of the strike, claiming that they were going back to work 'on humanitarian and professional grounds' and only on the condition that there would be no recriminations against anyone (*Herald*, 15 December, 1988). They warned, 'legislation in future should begin at grassroots level and all affected parties must be consulted right from the beginning' (*Herald*, 15 December, 1988).

The Health Institutions and Services Bill

In spite of the promises made by the government, none of the strikers' demands were met until after another strike in June 1989. The 1989 strike was triggered by frustration from unmet demands and the introduction of a new bill intended to give the Minister of Health power to control entry into the private medical sector and conditions under which private practitioners practice. The memorandum of the Health Institutions and Services Bill, 1989, stated,

> This Bill will provide for the registration of health institutions, that is, hospitals, nursing homes, medical laboratories, clinics and other buildings used for medical and paramedical purposes and will allow the Minister of Health to regulate the services and treatment provided at such institutions.

The Bill was intended for every health practitioner registered with the Medical, Dental and Allied Professions Council, but operating outside government and university institutions. Psychologists, chiropractors, natural therapists, and traditional health practitioners were also to be covered. The Secretary for Health was supposed to establish a register of health institutions which would be open to the public, and it was to become mandatory that every private health institution be registered and all registration applications were to be made to the Secretary for Health, but some would be referred onto the Minister for his decision. The Minister of Health would set out the terms and conditions of registration for each type of institution, providing regulations stipulating the standard of construction and location of health institutions and the essential equipment, staffing levels, keeping of records and submission of reports, functions of inspectors, and penalties for the contravention of the regulations. Applications for registration could be rejected for failure to meet the stipulated conditions, or if the Minister considered the registration of an institution as being against the public or national interest. In addition, the Bill gave the Minister of Health power to designate inspectors with authority to enter and inspect health institutions, their books and records, and any obstruction or hindrance of such inspection would be an offence. Those health institutions already in existence before the adoption of the Act were to be given six months in which to obtain registration. In addition, all private health institutions were to have a license renewable every year on payment of a fee and these licenses were to be clearly displayed in the institution.

There was widespread opposition to the proposed Act from various sections of the medical profession. ZMA announced that it had no objections to the maintenance of standards in health institutions, but strongly objected to control of the 'activities of doctors, dentists, psychologists and traditional healers' and granting the Minister of Health 'sweeping power without any reference to bodies of experts' (*Herald*, 18 May, 1989). ZMA claimed that the Minister's aim was to prevent consultant doctors operating in the private sector except from hospitals (*Herald*, 18 May, 1989). It further pointed out that inspection of patients' records and doctors' financial records was unethical.

ZMA claimed that many doctors were considering leaving the country and the Bill was likely to be a disincentive for foreign and local investors who prefer private medicine, which was already shrinking as a result of retirement and emigration. It queried whether Government had abandoned its policy of a dual health service, comprising the public and the private sector, enunciated in the 1984 White Paper on health. ZMA warned that the adoption of the Bill would

> ... certainly mark the end of the private sector in health care and a mass loss of doctors from the country. We believe the situation needs to be liberalized and opened so that doctors will be encouraged into this beautiful land of ours, not frightened away by unreasonable legislation. (*Financial Gazette*, 26 May, 1989)

The HDA criticised the amount of power which the bill invested in one man, 'the minister, to run the entire health service system of the country' and its potential for restricting private practice (*Herald*, 25 May 1989). The HPC was opposed to the bill, which it saw as usurping some of its powers and vesting them in the Minister of Health. In particular, it felt that the inspection, licensing and registration of the health services and institutions should be its own responsibility.

The Ministry of Health denied that the Bill was about controlling who worked where, arguing that it was meant to ensure public access to the highest standards of medical and nursing care and to 'discourage mushrooming of unregistered illegal backyard surgeries, nursing homes etc' (*Herald*, 19 May, 1989). In effect, the Bill was withdrawn from Parliament after the first reading by the Minister of Health because of widespread opposition by the medical profession (*Herald*, 25 May, 1989). One senior official in the Ministry of Health claimed in an interview that the Bill was 'shot down by doctors'. The doctors opposed regulation by the Ministry of Health because it was likely to be more effective than the HPC which has been described as a 'toothless bull dog' and which was dominated by doctors. The Zimbabwe Nurses' Association claimed in interview that, an inspectorate operating under the HPC would not be effective because of doctors' tendency to cover up for each other.

152

The defeat of the Health Institutions and Services Bill was the single biggest success of the medical profession's attempts to ward off threats to its autonomy by the government since independence. The medical profession had successfully rejected the government's right to control the individual doctors' right to go into private practice, where they located their office, and under what conditions they practised. The serious threat posed by the Health Institutions and Services Bill to the interests of the medical profession temporarily united its different sections which for the first time acted as a group with common interests. The doctors were successful in their efforts partly because senior politicians, including the state President, rely on private medical practitioners and, in addition, some senior members of the government were also practising privately, as mentioned earlier. The result was that the divisions and conflicts of opinion in the ranks of the political and administrative elite in respect of this legislation and the future of private medicine, became evident to the medical profession which fully exploited this to the full. There was also serious opposition from the private economic sector which is the financial backbone of the country's economy, whose executives and senior employees patronise the private health sector. The Government also lacked the moral authority to deny doctors the right to increase their income through hard work when some of its own Ministers were guilty of amassing wealth through corruption. The unity of the profession during this period made it a formidable group to fight against.

Prior to this, the voice of the medical profession had almost exclusively been that of the white sector of the profession, represented by the College of Primary Care Physicians. From independence up to this point, the ZMA was quiet, a function of the conflictual position in which the leadership of the organisation found itself. The formerly discriminated black doctors had an ambivalent attitude to the health policies of the government. Policies like free health care for the poor had greatly benefitted the ordinary Zimbabweans, as had the end of institutional racial segregation from which they as a group had benefitted. On the other hand, the Government's policy towards private medicine threatened the economic interests of the whole medical profession. At the same time, they could not forget the white doctors' privileged position under colonialism and their ideological and racially motivated opposition to the present Government. In addition, white doctors had access to political and economic resources from which black doctors were excluded, such as shares in private hospitals, support of the private media, international press and foreign governments, and the opportunity to settle and practice in other countries such as South Africa, New Zealand and Australia.

One of the main results of the defeat of the Health Institutions and Services Bill is that, up to August 1995, private medical premises are only inspected by the local government authorities concerned with compliance with the municipal zoning regulations when they are initially opened. There remains no inspection of private medical premises to assess their suitability for medical purposes; qualifications and adequacy of employed staff; adequacy of equipment; patients records and treatment practices. This is quite unusual in a country in which other institutions serving the public such as butcheries and small grocery shops are subject to strict registration, inspection and regulation. Some of the provisions of the abortive Health Institutions and Services bill were incorporated into the 1992 Medical, Dental and Allied Professions Act, which provides for the establishment of an inspectorate, but up to August 1995 the composition and areas of competence of the inspectorate had still not been determined. The amendment of the Medical, Dental and Allied Professions Act in 1992, was acceptable because its provisions were going to be implemented by the Health Professions Council rather than the Ministry of Health.

The withdrawal of the Bill was a humiliating defeat for the Minister of Health and his officers and the medical profession seized this opportunity to air its general dissatisfaction with the Ministry of Health as whole. Some members of the ZMA informed the media that they would join the junior doctors if they went on strike to push for their demands which had still not been met mainly because there were no channels for getting grievances addressed by government, other than through industrial action. Less than a week after this, in June, 1989, 300 hospital doctors came out on strike to press their demands for better working conditions. The strike affected all the central hospitals and patients were turned away from both Parirenyatwa and Harare Hospitals, as the consultants and expatriate doctors who were on duty only handled emergency cases and at Parirenyatwa, the only surgery carried out was for private patients. The Minister of the Public Service informed the strikers that their status as employees in an essential service precluded strike action and that the new conditions of service, which were awaiting the approval of the Treasury and the President's office, would not be conveyed to them unless they went back to work (*Herald*, 13 June, 1989).

The striking doctors refused to go back to work and the Minister of the Public Service invoked the Law and Order Maintenance Act and 77 doctors were arrested, while others went into hiding. At the same time, more than two hundred medical students started boycotting classes in support of the strike and consultants at Parirenyatwa and Harare hospitals strongly condemned the arrest of the doctors and pledged their support for them. Meanwhile, the HDA executive stated that doctors would not go back to work until they were outrightly informed about their new conditions of service (*Herald*, 16 June,1989). The media reported that patients were dying and others were suffering from lack of medical attention and the public blamed government while pleading with doctors to go back to work.

A lot of people were shocked that doctors had such low salaries (*Herald*, 15 June, 1989). Even the editor of the state-owned and controlled largest daily newspaper supported the case of the doctors, 'there can be no denying that the junior doctors have a genuine case requiring urgent attention. The initial walk out was itself the result of what they considered to be government's insensitivity to their plight' (*Herald*, 15 June, 1989). The Zimbabwe Congress of Trade Unions stated that it,

> neither condemns nor supports the strike, ... the length of time that has elapsed since the raising of the grievances ... suggests that the strike was justified ... six months was long enough for the state to come up with whatever package ... The state can not be excused for dragging its feet for so long. (ZCTU press statement, 16 June, 1989)

The College of Primary Care Physicians led a delegation to the state President's office to protest the treatment of the strikers by both the Ministry of Health and the police. A privately run newspaper suggested three courses of action for the Government: 'settlement of the immediate dispute; a more acceptable minister; and a commission of inquiry into the health services' (*Financial Gazette*, 23 June, 1989).

After four days of strike, the state President appealed to the strikers to go back to work and assured them that the package would be released soon, and also promised to personally intervene with the Attorney General to ensure that the charges against those arrested would be dropped. The doctors immediately went back to work, convinced that the President would not let them down. In the package which was released soon after, interns were for the first time given a call allowance of Z$110 for week day calls and Z$130 for weekend call duty, while those who could not secure hospital accommodation were given an accommodation allowance of Z$300 per month. The period of employment in a designated institution before a practising certificate could be granted was reduced from five to three years after internship. In addition, all government employed doctors got a salary increment and all those in grades higher than interns, were granted an annual professional allowance ranging between Z$10000 and Z$ 18000 to make up for the loss of the right to practise privately. The Public Service Commission made it clear for the first time that, 'no doctor shall engage in private practice unless granted that privilege by the Minister on the recommendations of the Public service Commission' (Ministry of Health Memorandum, 16 June,1989).

The Public Service Commission approved private practice by consultants for two afternoons per week after the times had been agreed with the medical superintendent, and then authorised by the Secretary for Health. The Ministry of Health had to establish monitoring mechanisms to enable the medical superintendent to detect and check any abuse, and anyone who contravened these regulations would be charged under the Public Service Misconduct regulations. Anyone granted the right to practice privately had to forego the professional allowance but expatriate doctors could not engage in private practice nor could doctors in managerial posts such as divisional, provincial and departmental directors as well as medical superintendents and district medical officers.

The 1989 strike was a historic land-mark for the government employed doctors in that, for the first time, they were given a call-duty and professional allowance and, for the first time private practice was authorised for consultants, even though no monitoring mechanisms have were ever put in place. Doctors and dentists were the only occupational groups in the health sector granted permission to practice privately on a part-time basis, all other health workers were prohibited, even when on leave. The package which they were awarded distinguished doctors as the most important occupational group in the health care division of labour and from that point on, there was instilled in the general public and the Ministry of Health, a belief that medical services would collapse if doctors went on strike. The state President had personally intervened in their case, thus further confirming their importance even though this undermined the authority of the Minister of Health, set a bad precedent for the future and went some way in confirming the label that the Minister was unfit for the post. When both the Minister of Health and his Secretary left their posts in 1990, most people believe that they were casualties of the strike and the abortive Health Institutions and Services Bill.

In a personal interview, the then HDA president informed me that his organisation's failure to secure a more favourable settlement after the 1989 strike had led to the decision by most doctors to leave the country, which many did without fulfilling their bonding contract. Some of them left for post-graduate training in developed countries, while others left for neighbouring countries such as Botswana and the South African homelands. The turnover of doctors from government institutions reached a record high of 39 per cent in 1991, giving rise to an acute shortage. After the strike, junior doctors successfully resisted attempts to post them to rural district hospitals because of poor social facilities; possible separation from families; lack of financial incentives and lack of opportunities for earning extra income (MOH & CW, 1991).

Consequently, in 1989, only 50 per cent of the medical posts in the outlying district health institutions were filled and, of these, less than ten were occupied by Zimbabwean doctors (Laing, 1989:5), thus forcing the government to rely more on expatriate doctors whom it had initially regarded as a stop gap measure while it trained its own doctors. In the early 1990s, the government was still experiencing problems deploying Zimbabwean doctors to these institutions, in spite of providing some inducements in the form of scholarships for post-graduate studies after a rural posting. Thus, the government, which frequently expressed its commitment to the rural-based poor, was forced to rely on expatriate doctors who have no knowledge of the people's culture and language, guaranteeing literally no communication between the doctor and his or her patients.

In 1991, the Minister of Health stated that doctors who had contravened the bonding contract would no longer be disciplined by government. An amendment of the Medical, Dental and Allied Professions Act in 1992 reduced the period which doctors had to work before obtaining an open practising license from three years to one after the two year internship. The problem of staffing rural health institutions is gradually improving, although about 54 per cent of district hospital posts and 89 per cent of mission hospital posts are filled by expatriates and only 167 of the 218 rural medical posts are filled (*Sunday Mail*, 5 March, 1995).

The appointment in 1990 of Doctor Stamps as Minister of Health, a staunch, white private practitioner and former president of the College of Primary Care Physicians, marked a distinct shift in government policy towards the medical profession and the private medical sector. His appointment would relieve the government of pressure from the private health sector. Moreover, his appointment, which coincided with the introduction of ESAP, would facilitate the government's cooperation and promotion of the private health sector. In addition to being kindly disposed towards the private sector, he is also consultative in his management style. For example, on presenting the Medical Dental and Allied Professions Act of 1992, he announced, 'I ... commend this document which has been fully discussed with the ZMA and in the majority accepted as progressive' (Hansard 1992, vol.18:5892). Previous Ministers of Health had all been strong ruling party stalwarts and, even though they were doctors by profession, they closely followed the government's ideological orientation and did not consult the medical profession in policy-making.

In a bid to increase the attraction of government employment, all doctors were given a salary increment of 40 per cent in 1992, which created a big salary gap between doctors as group and other professionals in the health sector and in the civil service in general. The professional allowance was replaced with a retention allowance for all doctors, except interns, and is equivalent to 50 per cent of the doctor's basic salary. Only doctors were given the retention allowance in spite of the fact that other health occupations such as technologists and occupational therapists have higher turnover rates, thus illustrating the dominance of the medical profession within the Zimbabwean health sector. The previous caveat which stipulated that government-employed consultants engaging in part-time private practice would not get a professional allowance was dropped even though they are still allowed to practise privately. In addition, heads of departments and consultants get an untaxed representation allowance amounting to Z$979 per month whose purpose no one could clearly explain.

Private Practice by Government-employed Doctors

Private medicine remains lucrative in Zimbabwe, with more than 50 per cent of physicians registered in the country practising privately on a full-time basis. Since independence to 1989, health insurance membership grew by 60 per cent (Loewenson, 1989). In 1985, it was estimated that private practitioners in Zimbabwe earned at least twice what government-employed doctors earned (Manga, 1988:1136), while a survey carried out in 1991 showed that some private practitioners earned as much as five times more

(MOH & CW, 1991). One university consultant stated in interview, 'I get in a week in my surgery what I earn for a whole month at the University and I am only working part-time in my surgery'.

The previous chapter showed how extensively all levels of government-employed doctors are engaging in part-time private practice, most of which is undertaken during working hours. The Comptroller and Auditor General (1995) indicated that some consultants spend as long as three months without appearing for duty in a government hospital where they are employed but are still paid a full salary and are never disciplined because government fears that they will just resign. One senior consultant pointed out,

> Some superintendents leave their jobs to go and practice during working hours and this is known by the Minister and Secretary for Health, but they just decide to turn a blind eye. How do you expect such a superintendent to discipline a junior when it is well known that they do not stay in their work themselves ... I am personally not convinced by the argument that the Ministry of Health is afraid to discipline doctors. I think there is lack of political will.

The medical superintendent of one central hospital was consistently given by all grades of doctors as an example of a senior official who flagrantly practices during working hours, and although the Ministry of Health knows this, it has not acted allegedly because he is a close relative of a very senior political figure. His behaviour has seriously contributed to the erosion of the authority and regulatory powers of the Ministry of Health administration and has gone some way in paralysing the regulatory mechanisms of the institution which he heads as one of his functions is to initiate Public Service disciplinary procedures. One senior Ministry of Health official argued,

> Post-independence connections with *chefs* [powerful political figures] have undermined the authority of those in charge ... For a medical superintendent to discipline a doctor he has to have a report from the consultant but, in most cases, both are not there to report the misbehaviour.

One of the effects of consultants' doing private practice during working hours and the inaction by the Ministry of Health is that most junior doctors, who are not supposed to practice privately, are doing so and very often during normal working hours. All the junior doctors interviewed said that they do locum work, stating that they make as much from this work as from their government salaries. When I asked about locum work, one SRMO replied, 'Yes I do. Everyone does it. Otherwise how would we survive?' Another SRMO admitted, 'Yes I do. About six hours every week. Owners of surgeries call you when they need help. Some advertise in the newspapers while others come to the hospital looking for doctors. I sometimes take leave to do locum work'.

A senior official with the Health Professions Council stated that he is aware that this is happening, but could not do anything about it as the Council only reacts to reported complaints and not hearsay. The lack of a comprehensive employment contract and the nature of the regulatory structures for health workers, are some of the main causes of indiscipline in the Ministry. One consultant declared, 'As long as government does not pay enough, doctors will do private practice ... government pays army generals enough so that they cannot be bribed by the enemy, so why not pay doctors enough so they do not do locum work'? Another consultant asserted that doctors are not the only ones neglecting their normal duties in pursuit of private economic activities, but that this has become characteristic of most professions in the country, including politicians, because everything is expensive and salaries are not adequate. She said that previously when she entered a ward, 'nurses used to ask me about patients' conditions or some work-related issue. Now they tell me they are selling a crocheted table cloth or something imported from South Africa'.

The Comptroller and Auditor General (1995) found that although there are work timetables in some departments, consultants do not adhere to them. One senior consultant informed me that he was opposed to timetables and maintained that when doctors cannot be located it is because they have no bleeps and not because they were doing private practice as assumed by most people. He argued,

> The health system is going to the dogs because people are concerned with the absence or presence of doctors rather than with their performance ... The administration does not know what it is doing. These are not clinicians. That is why. I do a ward round at a time that suits me ... The Ministry of Health expects us to be in outpatients, tea break at such and such a time but we do not work like that. We are everywhere at any time ... Ministry of Health officials have not worked in government hospitals of such capacity ... They worked as senior house officers and ... did a

poor job at that ... ended up in high positions in the Ministry not because of merit and experience, but because of political connections.

It is unlikely that a senior consultant who refuses to admit that private practice during working hours is rampant and disruptive to hospital functioning would report or even discipline his or her juniors. All the consultants interviewed had the same lack of respect for senior Ministry of Health & Child Welfare officials who were alleged to be incapable managers. The Comptroller and Auditor General (1995) stated that even though the Ministry is very aware of the indiscipline, officials are reluctant to act because doctors would simply resign rather than work in government. The Ministry's problems with consultants practising privately resembles that of the British NHS and its consultants. Although, British consultants have contracts with the NHS, these do not specify the minimum time that they should work and NHS officials adopt the same excuses as their Zimbabwe counterparts for failing to discipline errant doctors (cf. Yates, 1995).

The lack of employment contracts and effective monitoring and control mechanisms has given government consultants freedom to engage in private practice outside the hospital almost to the same extent as full time private consultants. Thus, contrary to the proletarianisation thesis, employment in bureaucratic institutions does not necessarily result in a loss of economic autonomy. In fact, salaried employment gives doctors prestige in comparison with their counterparts in private practice, who largely deal with minor illnesses. It enhances their attractiveness to patients, who perceive them as more experienced and at the cutting edge of new developments in their specialties. The findings of this book contradict Johnson's (1973) assertion that doctors in post-colonial countries have little opportunity to practice privately and, in fact, the deterioration of government health institutions makes the private health sector more attractive for paying patients. Moreover, permission to practice privately in Zimbabwe is not dependent on the patronage of government officials.

Private Beds in Parirenyatwa

When the Parirenyatwa Group of Hospitals was opened to everyone in 1981, government and university consultants were given permission to admit their own private patients to the hospital as an incentive to retain their services, but the maximum number of beds which they could use for this purpose was never specified. There have been allegations that these consultants are increasingly referring government patients to Harare Hospital which is overstretched and has poorer facilities in order to leave more room for their private patients at Parirenyatwa (*Sunday Mail*, 29 May, 1994).

In 1994, the Minister of Health, 'expressed concern ... and hoped that the debate would ... look at whether Government and university doctors should be allowed to practice privately and whether it would not interfere with their service to public patients' (*Sunday Mail*, 29 May, 1994). He mentioned that he was going to announce measures to 'curb the abuse' (*Financial Gazette*, 16 June, 1994), but up to the end of 1995, no serious discussion or action had been taken in spite of further and more damning evidence of abuse from the Comptroller and Auditor General's report (1995).

Mbuya Nehanda, the maternity wing of Parirenyatwa Hospital operated without government obstetricians, with 95 per cent of the patients being treated by their own private obstetricians, among them government and university-employed consultants (MOH & CW Technical Report, 1994). The government's excuse was that its salaries could not possibly attract full-time obstetricians but the operational status of Mbuya Nehanda became a source of controversy in 1993/94, when a Parliamentary Committee stated, 'Of great concern to your committee was the fact that private doctors were using the facilities at Parirenyatwa, such as Mbuya Nehanda and the wards in the main complex, for their private patients without offering anything in return' (Parliament of Zimbabwe, 20 February, 1993:21).

In response, the Minister of Health announced that Parirenyatwa Hospital would restrict private patients to wards C1, D1 and D2, which were originally set aside for them, while Mbuya Nehanda Maternity Hospital would allocate only 30 per cent of its beds for private patients (*Herald*, 10 June, 1994). Government and university-employed consultants vowed that they were not going to implement the Minister's directive and if government pushed them, they threatened to stop looking after SDF patients and doing other government duties. In a meeting with government and university consultants, the Minister informed them that 'government was willing to close down both Parirenyatwa and Mbuya Nehanda Hospitals if consultants did not rally to government's help in running the two medical wings' (*Financial Gazette*, 16 June, 1994). The Ministry of Health did not pursue the issue but employed two full-time obstetricians to take care of government patients in Mbuya Nehanda in 1995. Attempts to obtain the figures of SDF patients admitted to Mbuya Nehanda in 1995 were unsuccessful, but I was informed by both the medical superintendent and the public relations officer, that SDF patients were still considerably less than 50 per cent of the total number of patients admitted.

An additional obstacle to the admission of government patients to Mbuya Nehanda Hospital may be the long list of items which the patient is required to bring for the baby and themselves on admission. While a private patient may have little problems purchasing these items, which include night dresses and dressing gown, bedroom slippers for the mother and matinee jackets, napkins, etc for the baby, they represent a major expense for low-income patients. Lennox (1993) found that these lists are a distinct deterrent for low-income patients, and even though they could still be admitted to the hospital without them, they would feel ill at ease and reluctant to go there.

It appears incredible that for 14 years, a government that announced its commitment to equity in health and curtailment of the private medical sector, maintained its best and largest maternity hospital exclusively for private patients when a large number of low-income patients slept on the floor at Harare Hospital, less than 10 kilometres away. Mbuya Nehanda, which has 188 beds caters for 15 per cent of the maternity patients delivered at central hospitals, compared to 46 per cent for Harare Hospital with 180 beds (Comptroller and Auditor General, 1995:8 & 9). The lack of a clear policy on private medicine and monitoring mechanisms of government consultants' activities has given them considerable economic autonomy, which sometimes rivals that of full-time private practitioners. They have been able to engage in private practice in government hospitals, on government time, for a long period without any regulation. Thus, salaried employment in and of itself does not necessarily result in loss of economic autonomy but depends on the terms of the employment contract; the presence of monitoring and control mechanisms; whether or not there is prevalence of a culture of public accountability, as opposed to patronage; and the availability of a market for private practice in the society concerned.

The 1994 Doctors' Strike

Up to 1994, it appeared that the relatively powerful position which government-employed junior doctors occupied was unassailable and the government seemed willing to grant anything they asked for in order to retain their services. The 1994 doctors' strike provided me an opportunity, albeit an unexpected one, to assess the power of the medical profession in its struggle against the government. It also presented an opportunity for a critical analysis of inter- and intra-professional relations in the health sector.

In November 1993, the President of ZMA wrote a letter to the state President complaining about the deteriorating state of health services and asking him to personally intervene but this letter was forwarded to the Minister and Secretary for Health who called the ZMA executive for a meeting on 18 February, 1994. The ZMA executive in turn invited the President of HDA who brought a statement of hospital-based doctors' grievances which became the focus of the meeting.

In the document, the HDA asked for rent exemption for those living in hospital accommodation, a housing allowance of Z$1000 per month for interns living outside hospital accommodation, a Z$500 per month transport allowance for all interns, an increase of government car loans and lengthening of the repayment period , increase of call-duty allowance which was also to be tax free, removal of taxation on the retention allowance paid to middle rank and senior doctors, and a salary increase of 40 per cent for all government-employed doctors.

The Minister of Health explained that while he appreciated their grievances, most of the issues raised were the responsibility of other ministries over which he had no jurisdiction. He proposed that the HDA executive write a formal letter to his Ministry stating their grievances and the letter would be the basis on which the Ministry would then ask the Ministry of National Housing and Public Construction, the Ministry of Transport, the Public Service Commission, and the Ministry of Finance and Economic Development for a round table conference to discuss the grievances. The HDA did not do so but, instead, on 18 March, 1994, wrote a letter to the Minister of Health complaining about the lack of an official response on the grievances raised in the meeting, warning

> this apparent lack of interest in our affairs and sluggishness in responding to our documented grievances, ... is worrying in that it will inevitably culminate in a confrontational state. We look forward to your considered response within a maximum of 14 days. (HDA letter dated, 8 March, 1994)

The Principal Medical Director in the Ministry of Health replied by asking the HDA to follow the procedures suggested in the meeting of 18 February but also explained that since there was an on-going job evaluation exercise of all Government posts by the Public Service Commission, no review of conditions of service will be conducted for separate groups of civil servants until this exercise is over. It is therefore incumbent upon you and your association members to exercise restraint while a global solution is under urgent consideration. (PMD's letter dated 29 March, 1994)

On Friday, 15 April, 1994, 292 junior doctors comprising JRMOs, SRMOs, and SHOs, including those enrolled for post-graduate programmes at the four central hospitals in the country, went on an indefinite strike to push their demands. That Friday was the beginning of a long weekend which ended on 18 April, 1994, the 14th anniversary of Zimbabwe's independence and it was also the beginning of the school holidays and thousands of school children and urban workers were travelling to their rural homes for the long weekend. Choosing that weekend was intended to exert maximum pressure on the government, since such weekends are normally characterised by high rates of road traffic accidents and hospitals are normally very busy but the HDA executive assert, that doctors chose that weekend because as a group they felt they had nothing to celebrate and so they changed the previously agreed date of starting the strike from the 19 April, 1994 to 15 April, 1994. When it broke out, no warning of an impending strike had been given and the Minister and the Secretary for Health were out of the country on government business.

Negotiations were initiated that very morning, 15 April, and the acting Minister of Health who expressed sympathy with the strikers' grievances, asked them to resume work and promised that their grievances would be discussed after the weekend. The HDA negotiating team refused, insisting that 'in the past, we have been duped'. Even after a round table had been convened, the strikers refused to go back to work unless they had a definite written agreement.

When the negotiations recommenced, on 21 April 1994, the call allowance was agreed at the rate of 1.5 times for week day call duty and double rate for weekend call duty. Interns were given a housing allowance of up to Z$1000 per month and a block of 6 flats was reserved for interns. They were also awarded a transport allowance of Z$500 per month and the repayment period for new car loans was extended from 5 to 7 years. The loans for second-hand cars were to be reviewed upwards to match the going market prices and the department responsible for processing car loan applications promised to expedite junior doctors' applications. The striking doctors had secured all their demands, except the 40 per cent salary increment for all doctors which the government insisted could only be entertained after the job evaluation exercise. Thus, all the concessions secured only benefitted interns while SHOs (including post-graduate students) who were also on strike gained nothing, which not surprisingly, made them very unhappy with the package. Consequently, the HDA executive informed the Ministry of Health that the '40 per cent salary increase across the board is not negotiable' (HDA Executive Minutes, 21 April, 1994).

On 22 April, 1994, the Minister of the Public Service, Labour and Manpower Planning invoked Statutory Instrument 258 of 1990, according to which the Public Service Commission can order striking workers to go back to work and if they refuse to comply, it can summarily dismiss them (Statutory Instrument 258, 1990: 1582-1584). The Minister ordered the striking doctors to go back to work by 0800 hours the next day, 23 April, 1994 but the junior doctors refused and they were all sacked on 25 April, 1994. The Minister announced in Parliament and on national television that striking doctors had been given a package worth Z$90,000 per person per annum and yet still insisted on 40 per cent immediately. He declared that government was prepared to close the big hospitals rather than give in to the doctors and he maintained, 'there is no doubt that the measures taken were meant to nip the insolence in the bud and what was clearly a creeping in of anarchy' (*Herald*, 5 May, 1994).

Following the sacking of the doctors, all outpatients and antenatal clinics at the central hospitals were temporarily suspended and only patients needing emergency or critical attention could go there and these were attended to by army doctors, those employed in City Health departments, senior doctors and expatriate doctors. The Minister announced that those who wanted to resume work had to reapply to the Public Service Commission, as provided for in section 7(2) of Statutory Instrument 258 of 1990. On 27 April, 1994, all interns in government accommodation were served with a one month notice to vacate, and at the same time, interns were reminded of an HPC regulation which specifies that if internship is interrupted by a period exceeding a month, they have to serve an additional 6 months as interns. Although most SHOs and post-graduate students wanted to continue the strike, most interns wanted to go back to work, because they had gained the most from the strike, but also stood to loose the most from staying away from work longer. Others had pressing economic commitments for which they needed their May salary and if they stayed on strike much longer they would not be paid for the month.

The HDA executive and the media were informed that a number of application letters of re-employment had been received by the Ministry of Health. Fearing the collapse of the strike as more doctors applied to go back to work, the HDA executive advised its members to resume work with the gains they had secured, since they were unlikely to get any more. The HDA drafted a letter to the Public Service Commission stating that doctors had decided to go back to work 'on humanitarian grounds' and all of them signed a copy, but this was rejected and instead, every striking doctor had to sign an individual letter drafted by the Public Service Commission in which they had to acknowledge participation in an unlawful strike and undertake never go on strike again. The letter further stated that the strikers were going back to work on the conditions on which they had come out. By 13 May, 1994, everyone was back at work, but all those interviewed after the strike expressed their humiliation at the way things had turned out. One SHO said, 'I am angry and humiliated. I had to go and beg to have my job back ... I would not have reapplied but I still have ten days to go before I get an open practising license'.

The HDA emerged divided and with its ego bruised as one member of the HDA executive stated,

> Like any defeated party in a confrontation, you get some people who are unhappy and feel that the executive sold out. We lost. We did not win. There is no place for collective bargaining and there is no place for strike action for doctors and the HDA in this country. Striking is not an effective weapon. The feeling among some members is that HDA cannot change things for doctors. The only party that can change things is the government.

On the fate of the HDA, one SRMO concluded,

> no one would be convinced to attend a meeting to discuss another strike in the future ... Not with the way the strike ended ... We are divided anyway. The HDA executive have been complaining that they are fighting on their own without the support of the rank and file.

The behaviour of the doctors during the strike and the outcome of the strike lost the HDA and its members some support among the public and other members of the profession. One striking doctor stated that expatriate doctors in his firm were so outraged by the strikers' behaviour that they were not even talking to him. A senior consultant described the striking junior doctors as 'yobos' in interview with me.

The HDA executive was portrayed as immature, selfish, irresponsible, unreasonable and arrogant by the government and the revelation by the Minister of the Public Service that doctors had secured a package worth Z$90,000 per person would have convinced some members of the public struggling under ESAP that the doctors' reaction was unreasonable. The state controlled media did not interview doctors or represent their views like they did during the 1989 strike, when they were able to elicit public sympathy.

On its part, the HDA executive advised individual doctors to pursue individual strategies, like leaving government service for further training abroad and employment in neighbouring countries, although it was becoming clear that the alternatives for employment outside government were becoming limited and striking was partly a realisation of this. Some Zimbabwean doctors who worked in South African allege that the indigenous blacks there appear hostile to all those who went to work in the country before independence because they broke sanctions against that country and helped sustain the apartheid regime. That perception, and the level of violence in that country, now dissuades some Zimbabweans considering working there as a serious option. In addition, competition for jobs in South Africa is now intense as the number of applicants now includes doctors who would not work under the old apartheid regime. Before the world economic recession of the 1980s and the break-up of the former Eastern European block, Zimbabwean doctors could get scholarships to pursue post-graduate education in western developed countries but this option is now almost non-existent for most.

Similarly, although the private medical sector in Zimbabwe is still lucrative, it will undoubtably not be long before it gets saturated. In fact, some specialties are oversubscribed and there are already conflicts with general practitioners because consultants are not sending back patients referred to them after the original condition is treated (CPCP, 1992). Some of the junior doctors interviewed even alleged that high failure rates in some post-graduate programmes are a deliberate strategy by lecturers to limit competition in their specialties. Over 75 per cent of private practitioners in the country are located in Harare and Bulawayo, the two largest cities, and it is unlikely that there is much more room for expansion for the private medical sector. It is, therefore, possible that more doctors will, in future, remain in the public service. At the moment, there are a handful of specialists at Zimbabwe's provincial hospitals and none at district level, but some junior doctors indicated that they would not be averse to working at these hospitals if the accommodation was adequate and the rural allowance was reasonable. It is possible, then, that the strike has marked the beginning of a decline in doctors' economic autonomy, as most options become closed to them and as they seriously consider government employment as a life-long career option. Ministry of Health officials, could not hide their jubilation at the outcome of the strike as one of them stated in interview, 'Doctors have been posturing for years about how the system would grind to a halt if they went on strike, but this strike showed that they have no impact on health care at all'.

While the end of the strike was humiliating for the doctors who also lost half their May salary, this should not overshadow the amount of economic gains which they made from the strike. They emerged as the highest paid professional group in the whole government and, in fact, the gains totally distorted the salary structure of the whole civil service and of the medical hierarchy. The remuneration package for interns is now more than that of doctors several rungs higher than themselves as the latter lose their entitlement to call- duty, housing and transport allowances on completion of internship and receive the retention allowance instead.

The Ministry of Health did not escape from the strike unscathed, particularly as the general feeling was that the strike was due to poor communication between the Ministry and its employees. An acting Minister was able to secure doctors' demands in a week, which the real Minister had failed to do over a much longer period. The acting minister, a medical doctor, a long serving party member, a former Minister of Health, Secretary for Health in the Politburo and a powerful Minister in the government, and would be able to make a strong case to his equally long serving Cabinet colleagues. The Minister of Health, on the other hand, is a Presidential appointee to parliament, has been in government for a much shorter period than most, and does not sit in the ruling party's Politburo where Government policies are decided. The President's strategy of appointing a man influential in the private sector but with no political currency in the country was a brilliant move, in that it effectively silenced the normally vocal white medical lobby. On the other hand, even though the Minister of Health is a staunch supporter of the private health sector, the pillars of the Government's health policy are firmly in place and he can not derail them in favour of the interests of the private sector.

The strike highlighted the varied interests of the different sectors of the medical profession by hierarchical level, employment sector and race. Had all the different grades and sectors of the medical profession rallied behind the striking doctors, the Government could have been forced to award all their demands, but as it turned out, the strike highlighted the conflicting interests of the different medical factions and enabled Government to capitalise on the apparent divisions.

At the outbreak of the strike, the ZMA did not issue a statement, although its President told the media that his organization was 'indifferent' to the strike. In another context, he stated that his organization sympathized with the doctors' grievances, but that the decision to go on strike was that of the HDA and did not involve the ZMA. There was an outcry by some doctors in ZMA who distanced themselves from their President's statement but, nonetheless, did not offer an alternative position. When I asked about the relationship of HDA and ZMA, the HDA president explained that, except that they were in the same profession, there was 'no common ground' between the two organizations.

The reaction of the president of the ZMA was an indication of his displeasure at the HDA's failure to follow the procedures agreed on in the 18 February meeting with the Minister of Health. It is likely that the ZMA President felt that the junior doctor's strike jeopardised the new consultative stance adopted by the Ministry of Health, manifested in the meeting which had already taken place. This was a new and welcome development for ZMA which had up to then been almost totally ignored by Government in the determination of health policy since independence (ZMA Newsletter, 1992). The President of ZMA informed me that in his opinion, the Minister of Health appeared to be sincere and should have been given time to act on the issues raised in the document without the disturbance of the strike.

Government senior doctors and University consultants worked during the strike and did not, as in 1989, openly support the strikers or even threaten to join them. No members of the medical profession in Harare issued a statement on the strike and although some of the consultants supported the strike, they felt that junior doctors should have left emergency cover, while others did not support the strike on ethical grounds. Junior doctors stated that there was no need to leave emergency cover because consultants and registrars were not on strike and therefore could provide medical care, but of course this made it difficult for consultants to spend more time in their private surgeries as they would normally. The junior doctors interviewed felt betrayed by the consultants, but the irony is that they also gained from the strike, as they had more time to do locum work in private surgeries where business was more brisk than usual.

As discussed in Chapter 5, another less publicly discussed source of conflict between the consultants and the junior doctors is that of overwork of juniors as a result of consultants spending more time in their private rooms. Consultants supported the 1989 doctors' strike because the abortive Health Institutions and Service Bill affected the interests of the whole medical profession, whereas the issues which led to the 1994 strike largely applied only to junior doctors. It is also possible that the consultants, who have greatly benefitted from the *status quo*, did not want to focus attention on themselves by supporting the strike.

The strike also highlighted the differences of interest between the Zimbabwean and expatriate doctors who worked over-time during the strike, contrary to the expectations of the strikers. Some junior doctors stated that their attitude to the expatriates cooled after the strike even though the latter's contracts prohibit them from participating in industrial action. Their presence does go some way in reducing the bargaining power of Zimbabwean doctors because the government can always rely on them.

The College of Primary Care Physicians, which was very active on behalf of the junior doctors during the 1989 strike, did not even issue a public statement during the 1994 strike. Normally, it would clutch on anything that embarrasses government and would therefore support the strike action but this time, it is likely that CPCP did not because the Minister of Health is a former President of their organization. Supporting the strikers would have weakened the Minister's position and possibly cost him his government post and in fact, some private practitioners volunteered to help out at central hospitals in Bulawayo in the evenings when their own surgeries were closed. The lack of strong support for the strike from across the medical ranks considerably weakened the strikers' bargaining power and enabled government to take a strong stance against them.

Inter-professional Reactions to the Strike

The President of the Zimbabwe Nurses' Association wrote to the HDA president,

the nurses are behind you in your strike for better conditions of work ...
ZINA supports you and this is why we have decided to remain on duty
providing service to the patients ... As Sisters and Brothers committed to
service to Humanity, we pledge that we indeed support you and urge the
Ministry of Health to respond positively to your requests immediately.
(Letter by ZINA president to HDA president dated, 25 April, 1995)

The very next day, the president of ZINA wrote a letter to the state
President to inform him on the,

official stand the Nurses of Zimbabwe have taken as regards the strike.
The Nurses of Zimbabwe will not withdraw their labour in view of the
strike, but support hospital doctors in seeking better conditions of service.
We appeal to you as our Father to assist in resolving this matter. (Letter
by ZINA President to the state President, 26 April, 1995)

The nurses' letter to the state President reassured government that
the health service was not about to grind to a halt as would be the case if
nurses went on strike and this went someway in strengthening government's
resolve not to give in to the strikers. The nurses could work with the senior
doctors, expatriate and army doctors, and other volunteers to keep the
system going. At the same time, the Secretary General of ZINA told the
media that nurses were waiting for government to address the demands of
doctors before they forwarded their own. This latter statement was a veiled
threat to Government that it dare not give doctors another salary increment
and leave out everyone else in the health sector, as it had done in 1992. In
fact, the HDA executive and other striking doctors had hoped that nurses
would join the strike, although they did not openly say so. ZINA's reaction,
then was intended to strengthen the Government's hand during the strike
while at the same time ensuring that the Government owed the nurses a
debt. The nurses were rewarded by the creation of 400 new nurses posts in
government hospitals soon after the strike, after a long time of complaining
about shortage of nurses in hospitals.

Everything considered, ZINA's reaction was not totally unexpected
as it is one of the groups that is seriously challenging the power of the
medical profession in the health sector. Moreover, ZINA has not hidden its
resentment of medical dominance in the Health Professions Council, as will
be discussed in Chapter 7. ZINA was unlikely to jeopardize its good
relationship with the state President (whose late wife was its patron) to
support a group that it is fighting against in the Health Professions Council.

Laboratory technologists and technicians came out on strike in sympathy with the striking doctors, since the junior doctors based in Harare had gone on strike in sympathy with them in November 1993, arguing that they were not able to do their work without laboratory test results. The technologists and technicians who joined the doctors' strike were also sacked when the 296 junior doctors were sacked on the 25 April, 1994 and during that period, urgent diagnostic tests had to be sent to private laboratories. Radiographers, who joined the strike in sympathy with the striking junior doctors, were also sacked on 29 April, 1994.

Public prosecutors staged a sit-in and demanded an immediate audience with the Attorney General, who refused, and the Chief Law Officer informed them that they would be suspended if they did not go back to work because their action was illegal, and consequently, they went back to work after only one day of strike action. The Zimbabwe Teachers Association gave the government until the end of May to address its grievances and threatened, 'it will be difficult to restrain our members from striking' (*Sunday Mail*, 15 May, 1994). At the same time, customs officials also threatened to go on strike unless the government met their demands for higher salaries. Meanwhile, the Zimbabwe Congress of Trade Unions advised all workers not to accept pay settlements of less than 25 per cent from their employers.

The spate of demands by various sections of the civil service is likely to have hardened the government's resolve in dealing with the junior doctors. Under the circumstances, government could not be seen to be conceding to the junior doctors because it would have given the impression that strike action is effective, which would probably have resulted in wild cat strikes, as had happened in 1981 (see Sachikonye, 1986). However, concessions could be made on demands that are specific to medical work. The Secretary of the Zimbabwe Trade Union Congress points out that conceding to the doctors' demand for a 40 per cent increment would have '... created a ripple effect ... in the whole civil service' ([Medical Student] *Magazine*, 29 May, 1994). In June 1994, the government announced a salary increment for all civil servants ranging from 10 to 23 per cent which was effected before the job evaluation exercise was completed.

Other Health Policies with Potential to Reduce Doctors' Economic Autonomy

Free Health Care

As explained in Chapter 4, the government introduced free health care for those earning less than Z$150 in 1980. This policy could not affect the economic autonomy of doctors' with regards to their income from their government activities because their salaries are not linked to the number of patients that they attend to. It, however, had the potential of reducing the size of the private medical market from which they obtain some of their income, as pointed out earlier. It was assumed that more people would go to the hospitals where treatment was free than to private practitioners. Occasionally, before the introduction of this policy, even poor patients used to consult private doctors but they constituted a very small proportion of the private market, 90 per cent of which depends on health insurance schemes (MOH & CW, 1992). But as pointed out earlier, a number of people who did not legitimately fall into that category abused the system and were treated free, even though their impact on the private health market could have been equally negligible. We can, therefore conclude that the impact of the introduction of free health care was indirect and minimal if at all.

Legalization of Traditional Medicine

As mentioned in Chapter 4, traditional medicine was legalised in 1981 through the Traditional Medical Practitioners Act. I assumed that this would reduce doctors' economic autonomy as people could openly consult alternative practitioners and they, in turn, could use all of their diagnostic methods in their practice. But, in fact, even though traditional medical practitioners' activities had been severely constrained during the colonial era, about 75 per cent of the Zimbabwean population continued to rely on their services (Chavunduka, 1978).

No studies have been carried out to analyze the impact of the Act on the use of traditional medicine, but the terms of the Act itself did not grant the traditional healers much more than the right to practice without harassment and the right to self-regulation. Traditional healers have not been incorporated into the national health care system and therefore cannot offer their services in government hospitals. Moreover, since they are not recognized by health insurance organisations, those who consult them still have to pay out of pocket for services and are not reimbursed by the health insurance organisations. This means that unless the disease is seen as needing the services of a traditional healer, holders of health insurance policies are likely to consult Western trained doctors for economic reason. Patients who consult traditional healers still have to produce a certificate furnished by a doctor, which means that they still have to pay for that service.

Another reason why doctors' economic autonomy is not threatened by traditional healers is that, in fact, peoples' choice of type of health care is determined by their condition, i.e. whether the illness is defined as natural or unnatural (Bourdillon, 1987). Chronic, life threatening illnesses, and those which cannot be easily explained are regarded as unnatural are deemed to be due to an invisible cause and therefore needing the services of a traditional healer, a diviner who can communicate with the spirit world and identify the underlying cause (Bourdillon, 1987). On the other hand, acute conditions, including infections, are taken to the doctor or hospital.

A popular branch of traditional medicine which has been encouraged by government is that of traditional midwifery, which this is widely used in rural areas, but this does not threaten doctors' economic autonomy because those who resort to it are not likely to be able to afford the services of an obstetrician anyway. The activities of traditional healers do not have an impact on the economic autonomy of government-employed doctors as far as their government salaries are concerned and may have very little impact on their private practice market. Everything considered, we can conclude that traditional healers have little or no impact on the economic autonomy of government-employed doctors who have effectively retained their gate-keeping functions.

Conclusions

Government-employed doctors of all levels have more economic autonomy than their counterparts in Britain, for example. On paper their terms of employment are comparable but in reality, Zimbabwean doctors have higher degree of economic autonomy, largely because of: the lack of effective mechanisms for monitoring and enforcing those in place; a relatively large private medical sector and employment opportunities in neighbouring countries; a shortage of medical doctors in the country; cultural beliefs about the social and economic rewards befitting doctors; the dominance of medical doctors in the higher echelons of the Ministry of Health; and political patronage.

From the late 1980s, junior doctors have been able to force government to reverse policies that have a negative impact on the medical profession in the country, for example, reducing the period which they have to work in Government before they could go into private practice from seven years in 1988 to three years in 1992. Not only have they effectively used the strike weapon, but they have also threatened government with high turnover rates, forcing it to rely on more expensive and sometimes less suitable expatriate doctors. They have been able to push government to give them much higher salaries than other professionals and civil servants in government employment. Interns are supposed to rely entirely on their government salary and not engage in private work and yet they do locum work, some of it during working hours, and no sanctions are applied, even though the highest officials in the Ministry of Health know about it.

Middle rank doctors also enjoy considerable autonomy but not as much as the junior doctors and consultants, hence the high turnover. Consultants have considerable economic autonomy, partly because their government employment contract does not specify the minimum number of hours that they have to work, and the division of work between themselves and their juniors. Not only are they on relatively high incomes in comparison with other civil servants, but their contract allows them to practice privately and, in addition, they are also given retention and representation allowances. Their working hours are not monitored and most do carry out a lot of private practice outside the hospital during working hours and moreover, they are able to admit an unspecified number of private patients in Parirenyatwa Hospital and look after them on Government time while being paid private fees.

The inability of ordinary Zimbabweans to distinguish the different levels of doctors has enabled unregistered interns to practice privately without fear of being reported. This, coupled with the existence of unscrupulous private practitioners who are willing to engage unlicensed doctors in their surgeries, gives junior doctors more economic autonomy than should be the case at their level. The Government is partly to blame for allowing individual doctors to open private surgeries in more than one location like supermarkets, which can be staffed by anyone. Interns are hungry and because they are not registered, they can be paid less than the going rate and make money for the owner of the surgery.

The fact that senior officials in the Ministry of Health are medical doctors has gone some way to ensuring that the demands of government doctors are dealt with more sympathetically. The fact that senior government officials are in their positions at the pleasure of the state President and can be relieved of their post at any time engenders a tendency not to antagonise other sectors of the medical profession lest one finds oneself knocking on their door for employment. This explains the indulgent attitude in dealing with doctors and the government's ambivalent position on the future of private medicine.

The high turnover of Ministers and Secretaries for Health since independence has weakened the position of office holders, especially as there is a belief that messing with doctors will result in loss of office. For example, the Ministry of Health has had six ministers in 14 years, and all have been doctors including the first Minister of Health, an avowed socialist who was sacked from government after serving for just over one year. He suddenly found himself unemployed, without any source of income, and had no option but to go and practice privately and from then on he never stopped even when he was re-appointed Minister in another ministry. His case clearly illustrates the dilemma that faces most senior officials who are therefore unlikely to destroy their only viable safety net, private medical practice. In addition, the tendency of the state President to intervene publicly instead of leaving those immediately responsible, i.e. his ministers in charge, appears to have produced a culture of inaction as heads of institutions and departments fear burning their fingers in the course of doing their job. Government officials charged with maintaining discipline are also emasculated by the nepotistic tendencies of some political leaders. Consequently, medical doctors of all levels have been able to extend their economic autonomy because none of the Ministry of Health officials have been able to effectively enforce existing regulatory mechanisms.

The continued existence of a vibrant private sector has played a big role in giving government-employed doctors substantial economic autonomy. It provides alternative and more attractive employment for a large number who can afford to spurn government employment and, at the same time, forcing government to raise the wages of those remaining in public service in order to retain them. The opposition of the medical profession to some aspects of the government's policies has safeguarded the economic autonomy of government-employed doctors. For example, the intervention of the vocal white medical sector through the College of Primary Care Physicians during the 1989 strike. In addition, the close links between the medical profession and the private economic sector which threatened to disinvest in the country if there were no private health services partly forced the government to reverse its attitude towards private medicine in Zimbabwe. The government which is heavily reliant on foreign donations and loans to implement its policies, was particularly vulnerable to these threats as became evident with the withdrawal of the Health Services and Institutions Bill of 1989.

7 Regulation of Medical Education, Registration and Discipline

Introduction

This chapter analyses the degree and nature of autonomy which the profession has in the regulation of medical education, registration and discipline. Society granted the profession in the United States and Britain the autonomy to regulate itself in the nineteenth century on the understanding that this would be done effectively ensuring: that their training would equip them with the essential skills; that those registered would continue to practise competently; and that the profession would protect the public from malpractice by disciplining those involved.

The process of self-regulation can be both informal and formal but the former, which is most congruent with professional norms, has proved less effective in practise because of professional etiquette which inhibits disparagement or criticism of colleagues' professional skills (Rosenthal, 1995; Stone, 1980). Formal methods of self-regulation have been carried out by medical associations and quasi-governmental organisations like the GMC, but these have also proved less effective than desired by the public (Stacey, 1992). The former have been more concerned with advancing the welfare of the professionals than ensuring clinical competence, while the activities of the latter have been hampered by the composition of these regulatory organisations and their inability to make formal provision for monitoring clinical competence (Stone, 1980). The legal system, which provides another mechanism through which individual doctors can be held accountable for their activities, has proved deficient because: it is not equally accessible to everyone; the system acts after the damage has been done; the deterrent effect of compensation is reduced by the fact that in most cases doctors do not pay out of pocket, and because it can lead to defensive medicine which pushes up costs (Stone, 1980).

In the last two decades it has been widely accepted in the United States and Britain that the medical profession has failed to keep its end of the social contract of monitoring and sanctioning the quality of work and behaviour of its members on behalf of society (Gabe, Kelleher and Williams, 1994). The perceived inadequacy of medical self-regulation and escalating health costs, most from medical care, have resulted in a jaundiced public perception of the profession and increased calls for governments to regulate the profession (Bjorkman, 1989; Light, 1993).

Johnson (1973) asserts that the medical profession in post-colonial states has little autonomy in the regulation of medical education, registration and discipline which are controlled by a state department or a by semi-autonomous organisation which is answerable to government and not to the profession. Consequently, the doctors in those countries are more concerned with maintaining good relations with political and administrative patrons than with professional colleagues. Johnson argues that the professional associations which are supposed to spearhead self-regulation are weak and ineffective and have not established an ethical code, most simply adopting one from the former colonial rulers. Not surprisingly, the professionals have not internalised the values associated with their profession in Western developed countries (Johnson, 1972). An examination of the nature of medical autonomy in Zimbabwe will enable us to evaluate the validity of these assertions.

This chapter examines the range of structures concerned with regulation of the medical profession, starting with the main responsible body, the HPC, in terms of its structure, the composition and balance of power of the different groups represented in it, its role and that of other interests in the regulation of medical education, registration, and discipline, paying particular attention to the disciplinary structures, the role of the medical profession in those structures, the kind of behaviour that is disciplined and its effectiveness in the maintenance of discipline. The role of the Public Service Commission, as the body immediately responsible for the regulation of government-employed doctors is also analyzed in detail. The McGowan case is considered at length because it marks a historical watershed and at the same time, provides a good opportunity for evaluating the effectiveness of the official disciplinary machinery.

The Health Professions Council (HPC)

In Zimbabwe, the Health Professions Council (HPC) is the body ultimately charged with the responsibility for regulating medical education, registration and discipline, although it is not the only one. It is, however, the only body which can register health professionals, providing them with the necessary licenses to practise and it is also the only one that can revoke these licenses.

The HPC is a corporate body established by parliament and given power to regulate health professions under the Medical, Dental and Allied Professions Act of 1971 (Chapter 224). Unlike the British General Medical Council (GMC) which only regulates the medical profession, the HPC is a multi-professional body, rather like the Swedish Medical Responsibility Board, and regulates the 33 health professions registered with it. As in the case of Sweden, the size of the medical profession in Zimbabwe is relatively small, numbering no more than 2,000 members. The Council is made up of 27 members, ten of whom are appointed by the Minister of Health, with the other 16 elected in accordance with the terms of the Act (See Appendix 7.1). Most of the Council members are representatives of the major professional groups registered with it, but there are also two lay persons appointed by the Minister of Health.

The Medical Dental and Allied Professions Act (1971) provides for an allocation of money to the HPC by the legislature but, according to its Registrar, the HPC has not asked for money from Government for as long as he can remember, although he could not say why. It relies on annual subscriptions paid by professionals registered with it and other fees that it charges health education institutions for supervision of examinations and other services.

In order to carry out its duties, the HPC, which is supposed to meet not less than three times a year, appoints an Executive Committee which exercises its powers and functions. This Committee, comprises nine members, meets at least three times a year. The Medical Dental and Allied Professions Act also provides for the creation of Education Committees for the various professional groups; a Disciplinary Committee; and a Practising Control Committee (see Figure 7.1 for composition of these committees). The functions of these committees will be discussed in more detail in the relevant sections of the chapter.

The Balance of Power in the HPC

Even though the medical profession is much smaller than other professional groups registered with the Council, it wields a disproportionate amount of influence due to the dominant role that it played in the formation and development of the Rhodesia Medical Council, now known as the Health Professions Council.

The dominance of the medical profession in the health sector is reflected in the influential positions held by the medical profession in the HPC and in other health-related organisations. According to the authority structure of the Ministry of Health, the heads of district and provincial health authorities and medical superintendents, who are in charge of the overall administration of government hospitals, can only be medical doctors. The latter position has been justified on the grounds that doctors can only be answerable to another doctor for their clinical work. Since independence all Ministers of Health have been medical doctors, as have been the Secretaries for Health as have other holders of senior positions in the Ministry. Between 1988-1991, even the head of the Health Manpower Training and Development Section was a medical practitioner.

The proportion of medical doctors in the HPC has decreased as the number of professions registered with the Council has grown, but is still larger than that of any other health profession in the Council. Out of the twenty seven members of the Council, five are medical doctors, and both the president and the vice-president, who are elected from the twenty seven members of Council, are and have always been medical doctors. In the absence of the president and his vice, members of the Council select another medical doctor to preside over the meeting. In addition, two of the nine members of the Executive Committee are medical doctors and the President of the Council, a medical doctor, is the chairperson of every committee of the Council.

The influence of the medical profession in the Council also derives from the cultural beliefs of Zimbabwean society, which generally holds that doctors know better than other health professions and deserve more respect and status. One of the major arguments put forward by nurses demanding a separate nurses' council is that even if the clauses in the Act specifying that the president and deputy of the HPC have to be medical doctors is removed, it would not make a difference because no one would vote for a nurse to be president when there are doctors in the Council. One Ministry of Health official maintained in an interview with me, 'there is no nurse without a doctor'.

The dominance of the medical profession in the Council is now being challenged as other professional groups have expressed their dissatisfaction with the imbalance of power in the Council. The Zimbabwe Nurses Association asked for a separate Nursing Council, arguing that the balance of power in favour of doctors does not make it possible for other professional groups to make a meaningful contribution in the HPC; that in the whole of the Southern Africa region, Zimbabwean nurses are the only ones without a separate nurses' council; that nurses as a group make the largest financial contribution to the HPC, at more than 50 per cent of its total income, and yet this is not reflected in the amount of influence they wield there. It was ZINA which objected to the name of the Council, which up to 1985 was called the Medical, Dental and Allied Professions Council, arguing against being included in the label 'Allied'. As a concession, the name was changed to the Health Professions Council.

Since the mid-1980s, ZINA has emerged as the most well organised health professional group in the country. Nurses have benefitted tremendously from the patronage of the state President's late wife, who was the official patron of ZINA. Through her, it was able to get access to the President and explain the nurses' grievances directly. Although there are some minor internal divisions between registered nurses and state certified nurses, the nursing profession is more united than the medical profession.

Figure 7.1   Composition of HPC Committees

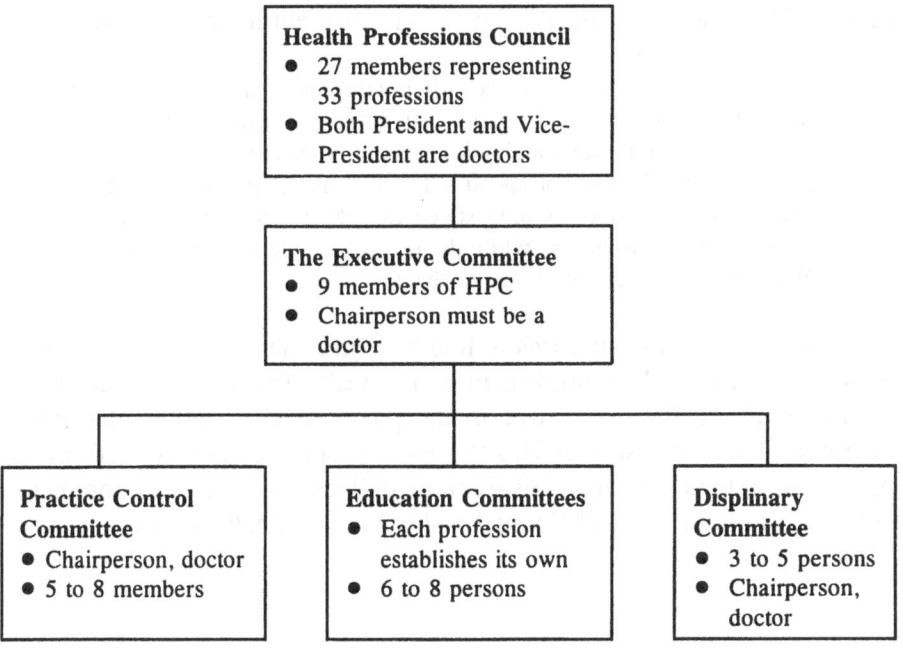

183

In 1993, ZINA submitted a Nurses Bill to the Ministry of Health and Child Welfare for presentation to parliament. The Ministry of Health refused to table the bill, after sitting on it for a year. In interview, the Minister of Health and Child Welfare declared that he would not sanction the creation of a Nurses' Council because everything that nurses asked for is being provided for in the proposed restructuring of the HPC. The President and the Registrar of the HPC on the other hand, pointed out in interviews that they are not opposed to a Nurses Council in principle, but feel that withdrawal of the nurses' financial contribution would cripple the activities of the HPC which was aiming to set up an inspectorate to check on the activities of registered members and the operations of health institutions, both which require money.

In the new structure of the HPC proposed by the Ministry of Health, each of the major professional groups registered with the HPC has its own semi-autonomous council, with the existing Council as the hub of the new structure. Each profession would have its own committees responsible for various functions, but reporting to the main Council on the occasions that it meets. There would be a central administration handling finances. Nurses feel that the new structure would not be effective in terms of regulating professionals who could still cover up for each other in the semi-autonomous councils. In an interview one HPC member representing the nurses insisted,

> Creation of separate councils will not increase the Council's ability to control the doctors. Even now, all cases are dealt with in individual professional committees and only the summaries are brought to the Council and we normally do not spend a lot of time on individual items. In the McGowan case, doctors only stated that the charge was that he failed to follow some procedures, while the doses he gave were not above normal. What could the rest of us say to that?

From the above discussion, it is clear that there is a challenge to the dominance of the medical profession in the Health Professions Council, but because of its position of power in the policy-making and implementing structures of the Ministry of Health, and the socio-cultural beliefs of the political elite, the challenge is likely to be deflected and medical dominance maintained in both the new Council and within the health sector.

Regulation of Medical Education

This section examines the role of the medical profession in the regulation of medical education in Zimbabwe. What roles do other interested parties and institutions play in the regulation of medical education? Who controls entry qualifications, the size of the medical school intake, the type of curriculum adopted, and the conditions of internship?

In Zimbabwe, the main parties in medical education are the University of Zimbabwe, which has the only medical school in the country; the Ministry of Health and Child Welfare, which is the largest health provider in the country; the professional associations; and the Health Professions Council. The policies adopted on the different aspects of medical education reflect the relative influence of these different parties, making decision-making in medical education potentially conflictual since these bodies have different expectations and interests. However, the level of conflict is reduced by the dominance of the medical profession in the decision-making machinery within each of the interest parties and institutions involved.

Conflict usually centres on determining the quantity and quality of medical graduates (Freidson, 1988). The medical profession, through its associations, is interested in ensuring that decisions taken on medical education do not devalue the profession and erode its economic position and bargaining power. In these terms, it is interested in both the intake to medical schools in order to avoid oversupply of doctors, and the type of curriculum adopted. A shortage of doctors is preferable to the medical profession because it increases the bargaining power of the profession for those employed in the public sector and limits competitiveness in the private medical market.

Gish (1971) states that the main area of conflict is over the type of curricula adopted because in most former colonies they were modelled on those of the colonial power. On coming to power, most post-colonial governments prefer a curriculum suitable for the disease patterns of the majority of the people in the country (Gish, 1971; Gish and Martin, 1979), and for that reason, the colonial curricula are almost always unsuitable. Developing countries are concerned with infectious diseases such as tuberculosis, measles, and, more recently, AIDS, as well as other diseases such as malnutrition which result from poverty, which do not need technological intervention. On the other hand, developed countries have to deal with degenerative diseases such as hypertension, heart disease and cancers and their medical curricula are tailored to suit those conditions. However, the medical profession clearly prefers a curriculum which is internationally acceptable and a health system which keeps up with the latest developments in health care for fear of being 'cut off' from the international fora of medicine.

For the same reason, training abroad and affiliation to professional associations in developed countries fosters expectations that are not appropriate for health services of a developing country. These expectations are shared by those trained locally because of the influence of their lecturers, almost all of whom have been abroad where they have gone through the process of medical acculturation. The conflict of interest is even more significant for the policy-makers who are largely doctors and have to decide what is right for the profession and for the country. Usually the profession wins under the guise of maintaining professional standards. An internationally acceptable curriculum is unsuitable as it makes migration inevitable because the declining economic performance of many developing countries does not allow salaries to match those of developed countries (Gish and Martin, 1979). To forestall this, governments attempt to retain doctors by offering them high salaries, which not only reduces the numbers which a government can employ, but also results in gross inequality in domestic income distribution.

The Ministry of Health and the Professional Associations

As pointed out in Chapter 4, the post-colonial government expressed the desire to see changes in both the quality and quantity of medical graduates. The Minister called for the doubling of the medical school intake, which was implemented in 1981. The government's call for a more relevant curriculum was also heeded by the University Medical School. The reviewed curriculum adopted in 1985 incorporated most of the government's suggestions.

The medical associations did not react publicly to the Government's call for an increased medical intake and change of curriculum because, as pointed out in Chapters 4 and 6, they were not very active in the early 1980s. In interviews, senior doctors remarked that they could not remember a single dissenting voice on most of the policies proposed by the government and some medical lecturers claimed that they actually wrote some of the Minister's early speeches. But more importantly, they are all members of a small professional group and tend to liaise with each other in public houses and other social venues. One former senior policy-maker whom I asked about the potential conflict of interests between the profession and government policies neatly summed up the sentiments shared by most of them, 'I am a doctor first, foremost and last'.

The Health Professions Council and the University Faculty of Medicine

The Health Professions Council, as the only body in the country that registers medical practitioners and issues them with practising certificates, has the responsibility to ensure that those who are registered have received a suitable education. The Medical Dental and Allied Professions Council Act (1971), provides for the creation of education committees to

> advise the Council on any matter of education in the field in respect of which it is established; and to satisfy itself and the Council that the curricula in every teaching institution ... are such that graduates will have a sufficient basic knowledge for the practise of their profession or calling. (Medical, Dental and Allied Professions Act, 1971:20)

The education committee for the medical profession is comprised of medical doctors only, but includes others from outside the HPC.

The education committee can, with the authority of the Health Professions Council, appoint 'inspectors to visit the university, hospital or other institution or premises where instruction is given to or examinations conducted for students who intend to apply for registration in terms of this Act (Medical Dental and Allied Professions Act, 1971:20). The Council, therefore, has responsibility to ensure that all the different aspects of medical education are satisfactorily met. The Act does not spell out the HPC's role in determination of entry qualifications and size of classes, although the University medical school curriculum is approved by the HPC; and reports of the external examiner on medical examinations are sent to the HPC.

The Council is advised by the Medical Education Committee on the position that it takes on the different aspects of medical education. As the President of the Council is always from the medical school his or her opinions are likely to reflect those of the medical school. This means that there is not much conflict between the HPC and the Medical School and the final decisions ratified by the Council reflect the views of the medical school lecturers and the Ministry of Health.

Medical education in Zimbabwe is offered by the University of Zimbabwe, an autonomous body created by an act of parliament in 1956. The university's financial requirements, including lecturers' salaries, are met through a block grant from central government through the Ministry of Education and almost all university students receive loans from the government for their university and subsistence fees. The university's position reflects the views of the medical school because of the assumption that medical lecturers know more about medical education than anyone else. The government is the single largest employer of medical practitioners and the medical school accepts that the government should have a say in the type of doctor that it requires. The beds, patients and all the facilities essential for clinical education belong to the government and internship takes place in its hospitals.

Entry to the University of Zimbabwe medical school exclusively depends on 'A' level results and the university simply decides the number that can be comfortably accommodated in the school and the applicants with the best results are taken until that number is reached. Since the doubling of the medical school intake in 1981, the government asked that the medical school intake be increased but the University consistently refused, pointing out that the physical facilities and equipment could not exceed an annual medical intake of 80 students. One of the spin-offs of the 1994 doctors' strike was that the Government granted the University Z$97 million to put up the necessary buildings. Accordingly, the medical school intake was doubled again in 1996 to 160 per annum. Clearly, the main decision-maker on the size of the medical school intake is the government because of its control of finance for student grants, lecturers' salaries and provision of the essential buildings and equipment.

The tradition of medical education established under the University of Birmingham is one which the medical school remains proud of today. The objective of the first medical curriculum, used with minor changes from 1963 to 1985, was to train doctors whose qualifications were recognised locally and overseas where some of the graduates would choose to work or undertake postgraduate education.

In interviews, medical lecturers expressed their pride in the fact they were producing doctors who were performing very highly in both South African and British post-graduate examinations and considered suitable for employment in those countries. The measure of suitability and quality of education is eligibility for employment in countries more developed than Zimbabwe, rather than ability to deal with local conditions. This clearly illustrates the dilemma which faced the new government in the implementation of all its policies in health and other sectors. It espoused

188

socialist policies, but relied on personnel trained in western capitalist countries to implement them.

The Medical School was last inspected in 1977 by an international committee, and in spite of changes of curriculum, doubling of the undergraduate intake, lengthening of the internship period, and the introduction of many post-graduate courses, no inspection of the school for adequacy of equipment and teaching staff has been undertaken. According to the conditions laid down when the medical school was first opened, interns are supposed to be under constant supervision and should care for a maximum of 25 patients and no less than 15. The Medical Education Committee of the HPC is, among other things supposed to 'satisfy itself as to the training duties and facilities for experience for interns where applicable' (Medical, Dental and Allied Professions Act, 1971:20). However, this has not been done since independence, even though complaints have been raised about the lack of supervision and teaching, and about overwork. It is common knowledge, as discussed in Chapter 5, that interns are engaging in locum work, in clear violation of the conditions on their practise certificates, and yet both the Practise Control Committee and the Medical Education Committee have not acted on this.

Many Diploma and Masters degree programmes in radiotherapy, medicine, surgery, psychiatry, paediatrics, obstetrics and gynaecology, anaesthetics, and ophthalmology were introduced after independence in 1980 with the aim of meeting the needs of the country for specialists and those of medical graduates for post-graduate qualifications. Because these specialist courses are not recognized internationally, some of the students leave in the middle of their courses for South Africa or Western developed countries for postgraduate training which is internationally recognised and marketable.

Postgraduate education has been compromised by the shortage of lecturers and the poor teaching input by those in the departments who are accused of spending more time in their private surgeries at the expense of teaching. The Director of the Institute of Continuing Health Education, University of Zimbabwe, described the students and their lecturers as 'part-time students and part-time lecturers' due to the inadequate amount of work which they put into postgraduate education. With all these problems, it is little wonder that these programmes have had high drop-out and failure rates. For example, the failure and drop-out rates from Paediatrics and Psychiatry for the years 1989 to 1991 was over 50 per cent, while that in General Medicine was over 80 per cent, and in Obstetrics and Gynaecology 35 per cent (Comptroller and Auditor General's Report, 1995:54).

When I asked senior HPC officials why no inspection of the school has taken place since 1977, I was informed that inspection is only done on request, or if a complaint is lodged concerning the quality of teaching, but apparently even the external examiners have not complained. The HPC should, in fact, have initiated an inspection of the medical education programme in the wake of the doubling of the medical school intake, alongside reviews of the curriculum, the introduction of so many post-graduate courses, and in the face of so many complaints concerning internship and post-graduate education. We can conclude that the HPC has failed to effectively regulate medical education as prescribed by the Act governing it. The dominance of the medical profession in all the institutions responsible for regulating medical education has ensured that no action is taken because the *status quo* is favourable to their individual and corporate interests.

Registration

The rationale for the HPC overseeing medical education is to ensure that those placed on its registers have attained an acceptable level of competence. The Health Professions Council is the only body responsible for registering doctors and other health professionals and for that purpose it has a number of registers for the purpose of registering medical practitioners, comprising: the house officers' register for interns; the permanent register for all Zimbabwean doctors who have completed their internship; and the provisional register for expatriate doctors.

The HPC has the power to establish a Practice Control Committee (PCC) whose main function is to evaluate applications for entry into the various registers. The PCC is chaired by the President of the HPC and comprises between five and eight members appointed by the Council. As stated earlier, it has the power to appoint inspectors to enter any health institution at any reasonable time, to question any employees at the institution, and to inspect its records if it is reasonably necessary for the detection of any offence with regard to a person's practising certificate. To date, the Committee has restricted its activities to the issuing of practising certificates for local graduates and vetting the qualifications of foreign graduates who apply individually to work in the country.

In the early 1980s, most expatriate doctors were recruited from English speaking Africa and western developed countries, particularly the

United Kingdom. There were no problems because the curricula were comparable to that of Zimbabwe, but by the mid-1980s, the Government had become dependent on doctors from the former Eastern European countries and the Indian sub-continent, who are faced with either unemployment or lower salaries in their own countries. Most of these doctors come on government-to- government agreements and the HPC can usually not assess the suitability of their qualifications because once the agreement is reached it has to accept them or risk embarrassing the Zimbabwean government and spoil relations with political allies. In interviews I was informed by some HPC officials that in a few cases, the Council has been forced to register and sanction the employment of doctors that it considered unsuitable.

One senior Ministry of Health official explained that some of these 'friendly' governments presented candidates who could speak English for interviews with visiting Zimbabwean officials who made the selection, but, in a number of cases, the doctors who finally turned up to work in Zimbabwe were different people who could not speak English. In 1995 it was revealed that one such bilateral agreement provides for the employment of eight doctors on three year contracts and they are all supposed to work together because of language problems (Comptroller and Auditor General's Report, 1995).

One HPC official mentioned a case in which the Council thought a whole group that had arrived in Zimbabwe was clearly unsuitable for employment and conveyed this to the Ministry of Health but, when the Ambassador of that country was informed, he warned the Zimbabwe Government that if they were repatriated, his country would cut technical assistance to Zimbabwe. These doctors were then employed on full salary but put in hospitals where they had to be supervised. Again, the Council had to abandon its usual registration criteria for political expediency. On the whole, the HPC is viewed as capable of screening expatriate doctors effectively if it could be left to make decisions on its own. We could conclude that in the registration of locally trained doctors, the Council has autonomy but its autonomy in the recruitment and registration of expatriate doctors is compromised by the political considerations of the government.

The Practise Control Committee has not established an inspectorate to carry out its other responsibilities, such as ensuring that those registered with the HPC are practising in accordance with the conditions on their licensing certificates and that all practise competently. In the absence of an inspectorate, a practitioner can continue to practise incompetently as long as they are not caught. The only way in which the Council may know about breaches in the standard of competence is if someone complains and, even then, the performance has to be grossly incompetent before the Council will apply sanctions on the accused. Monitoring to ensure competence to practice is also a thorny issue in other countries, such as Britain where the GMC has also not devised an adequate system (Rosenthal, 1995; Stacey, 1992).

Discipline

Government-employed doctors, who are the main focus of this study, are, like all other government employees, regulated by the Public Service (Disciplinary) Regulations 1992. They are, however, also regulated by other mechanisms which include medical associations law courts and parliament.

The Public Service Disciplinary Machinery

Government-employed doctors are regulated by a long chain comprising the firm structure, hospital management, the Ministry of Health and Child Welfare, and ultimately by the Public Service Commission through its Public Service Disciplinary Regulations. As mentioned earlier, these doctors are also subject to regulation by the HPC and a number of other regulatory structures.

Public Service Disciplinary Regulations supposedly deal with the following offences:

> absence from duty, including any abuse of sick leave without good cause; improper, negligent, inefficient or incompetent performance of duties; failure to perform any work or duty properly assigned, failure to obey lawful instruction ... improper, threatening, insubordinate or discourteous behaviour ... during the course of duty towards any member of the Public service or member of the Public ... unbecoming or indecorous behaviour including the consumption of intoxicating liquor and drugs to excess at any time or place in any manner or circumstances likely to bring the Public Service or any part thereof into disrespect or disrepute; ... failure to report improper conduct on the part of any member of the public service; practising nepotism or any other form of favouritism ...; undertaking or engaging in any other employment or service for remuneration without the written consent of the Commission. (Public Service [Disciplinary] Regulations, 1992:446-447)

The Zimbabwean health service does not have a separate regulatory structure specially created to deal with medical and other health workers in public hospitals, as is the case in England and Wales, and Sweden. The Public Service Disciplinary Regulations are supposed to cover all cases of misconduct in any government department regardless of the nature of its functions. The offenses listed in the Public Service Disciplinary Regulations do not include those arising from clinical practice and consequently, some of the offences which constitute clinical and professional misconduct in the health care context are not outlined, which means that behaviour that can have serious consequences for patients is dealt with inappropriately and leniently. For example, absence from work for office-bound civil servants rarely has fatal results, but on the other hand, absence of a doctor from work can have fatal results for his or her patients.

Mechanisms for Monitoring and Detecting Misconduct

According to the Public Service Disciplinary Regulations, if misconduct is suspected, the head of the station (in the case of doctors, a medical superintendent) is supposed to investigate the case and request the accused person to disclose all the necessary information within fourteen days. If the medical superintendent concludes that there has been misconduct, he or she informs the defendant of the allegation in writing and the latter also responds in writing and all this is forwarded to the Ministry of Health within seven days. The Head of the Ministry in turn, forwards the case to the Public Service Commission within seven days after adding his or her own comments on the case. The Public Service, on receiving the case, can ask that further investigations be carried out and the accused is allowed to respond to the findings of the investigation. A medical superintendent has no authority to discipline a doctor, but can suspend in cases of mental illness.

For the medical superintendent to initiate disciplinary procedures as head of the institution, he or she has to have information that an act of misconduct has been committed. He or she has to receive the information either from consultants as heads of medical firms, ward sisters, other health workers, or patients. The medical firm structure, which is an important mechanism for monitoring professional and clinical conduct, is not operating efficiently, as pointed out in Chapter 5 and, consequently, many acts of misconduct go undetected. The mere presence of a consultant deters perpetration of acts of misconduct by subordinates and, in addition, the

193

possibility of getting a bad report or failing a rotation is supposed to make doctors more conscientious in their work as all bad medical practices and unprofessional conduct are recorded in the doctor's file (Stacey, 1992). The consultants can only give accurate reports if they spend time with their juniors, but as we have seen, some of them spend considerable periods of time without doing so, consequently the reports do not necessarily reflect the performance of their subordinates. The Comptroller and Auditor General's report (1995) noted that some consultants indiscriminately give good reports to their subordinates and even the worst doctors are awarded 'very good' reports, thus removing the role of the report as a source of reliable information, a deterrent and a sanction.

The consultants that I interviewed stressed that before independence medical superintendents had authority and that being summoned before them was regarded with great trepidation by all. Apparently, one could get a severe reprimand from the medical superintendent for getting a bad report, failing a rotation or committing an act of misconduct. Within the hospital structure itself, rotation from one specialty to the next was not automatic as is the case now, but one had to apply to the head of the firm which one wished to join and if one had a bad report, one would experience problems getting accepted in the preferred firms.

Another mechanism which could assist in the detection of mistakes is medical audit, discussed in Chapter 5, but as pointed out, it is ineffective for detecting and controlling clinical mistakes as it operates in the Zimbabwean context. It is flawed by lack of institutional support and by the fact that it is voluntary, unsystematic and more concerned with the process rather than with patient outcomes and effectiveness.

The medical superintendent can also learn of acts of misconduct from nurses, but they cannot always detect clinical mistakes. One senior nursing officer mentioned in an interview that while she used to report drunk doctors and rude nurses, she no longer does so because often nothing is done and she loses face with her subordinates as she stated that before independence, she could tell a drunk doctor to get out of her ward but she can no longer do this because she does not have the same authority as she did then because her subordinates can appeal to persons in higher positions than herself with whom they may be related and the case can be squashed at any stage. In addition, even if a report is made, the Public Service Commission often concludes that the act of misconduct was due to inexperience and that the defendant should be given a chance to acquire experience.

A serious problem arising from the lack of special consideration of the nature of work in government hospitals is the lack of properly laid down channels for patients and aggrieved relatives to lodge complaints. As a result, complaints from the public about government health workers go all over the place and not always to the medical superintendent who is supposed to initiate Public Service disciplinary procedures. Some are directed to the ward, some to the medical superintendent, others to the Ministry of Health while others still are directed to the HPC. Consequently, a lot of patients' grievances are not addressed because of poor communication channels. In 1995, the Ministry of Health established a public relations office at Parirenyatwa Hospital to deal with any complaints arising there, but its effectiveness has yet to be assessed. The Zimbabwe Ministry of Health is in the process of establishing a Patients' Rights Charter to inform the public and patients about health services; the kind of behaviour that they should expect from health workers; and the channels for lodging complaints. While this is a big step in the Zimbabwean context, the reported acts of misconduct which proceed beyond the public relations officer are still supposed to be dealt with through the cumbersome and fairly ineffective Public Service Disciplinary procedures.

The sanctions at the disposal of the Public Service Commission when a charge of misconduct is successfully lodged include: discharge from the Public Service; forced resignation; denial of promotion; reduction in salary; and transfer to another department. In interviews with Ministry of Health and Child Welfare officials, medical doctors and other health workers, it emerged that doctors are rarely disciplined by the Public Service Commission because their cases are rarely reported. After reviewing the disciplinary machinery in government hospitals, the Comptroller and Auditor General (1995:30) concluded that there 'is no structure of punishment in government hospitals'. Although this is not entirely true, the ineffectiveness of the existing structures almost makes the statement true. There is for example, no coordination of the Public Service disciplinary structures and the HPC and hence, it is not clear at what stage in the long Public Service disciplinary procedures the HPC is supposed to be informed, and by whom. Consequently, even in cases of gross incompetence, government-employed doctors are rarely disciplined by the HPC, which has the ultimate weapon of removal from the register. It is therefore not surprising that the HPC receives most of its complaints and disciplinary cases from the very small proportion of patients treated in private hospitals. This is paradoxical because the government patients who are fairly uninformed and unassertive need the support of more effective disciplinary structures than those treated in private institutions who can sue or change doctors and hospitals.

The lack of clear channels would be less worrying if there was little evidence of indiscipline in the hospital but, in fact, health workers and the Comptroller and Auditor General stressed that the levels of indiscipline had increased considerably since independence, largely due to nepotism and lack of political will by those charged with the responsibility of maintaining medical discipline.

The Medical, Dental and Allied Professions Act (Chapter 224) and the HPC

The Medical, Dental and Allied Professions Act gives the HPC the responsibility to regulate all health workers registered with it regardless of their employment status. The Act defines the kinds of behaviour for which health workers registered with it can be disciplined; the composition of the disciplinary structures; the disciplinary procedures themselves; and the sanctions at its disposal.

Acts of misconduct for which medical doctors can be disciplined by the HPC
The HPC has the responsibility for disciplining a registered person who has been guilty of 'improper or disgraceful conduct' according to that profession or is 'grossly incompetent or has performed an act pertaining to his profession or calling in a grossly incompetent manner' (Medical, Dental and Allied Professions Act, 1987:42). However, the handbook, *Health Professions Council Functions and A Guide to Ethics*, states that the competence of the Executive Committee is not limited to offences defined by the practitioner's professional code of conduct in determining what constitutes improper or disgraceful behaviour, but does not elaborate on the other offences that it considers.

Other offences for which HPC can initiate disciplinary action in accordance with the Medical Dental and Allied Professions Act (1971) include: practising without a valid license; failing to notify the registrar of a change of address; practising outside conditions endorsed on one's practising certificate; and failure to implement Statutory Instrument 93 of 1993, discussed in Chapter 5. In addition, anyone convicted in a court of law is supposed to be referred to the HPC so that it can determine whether the crime constitutes improper, or disgraceful, or grossly incompetent behaviour.

Evidence so far suggests that the Executive Committee only refers to the Disciplinary Committee those cases which it considers to constitute improper, disgraceful or grossly incompetent behaviour. Other serious medical offences which are not judged as falling into this category are not sanctioned and this leaves the public unprotected from a considerable number of medical offences which may not fall into this category and yet can be equally fatal for the patient. The high threshold of what is defined as 'meriting disciplinary action' is comparable to that in Britain where the GMC is concerned with 'Serious Professional Misconduct', although the GMC has been debating changes in this respect for a number of years (Stacey, 1992). In Sweden, on the other hand, the Medical Responsibility Board (MRB) considers most complaints brought before it and does not limit itself to serious offences only. It also takes disciplinary action in cases concerning lack of consideration and respect in communicating with a patient and their family and for giving inadequate information to the patient and their family, in addition to dealing with more serious malpractice cases.

One serious problem in the determination of what constitutes improper and disgraceful conduct and gross incompetence by the HPC is that, according to the *Health Professions Council Functions and a Guide to Ethics* handbook, the HPC goes by what is currently accepted as ethical by the occupational group in question (HPC, 1993), but the HPC has not made it mandatory for every profession to have an ethical code. Consequently, most professions registered with it, including the medical profession, do not have ethical codes, likening the operations of the HPC in this ethical vacuum to that of a police force without the law to guide it. Whether a case has been passed on from the courts, has emanated from implementation of Instrument 93 of 1993, or from patients, the HPC faces the same dilemma of being unable to determine what is ethically acceptable to a profession. The seriousness of this omission became evident during the McGowan case when the medical profession could not agree on the ethicality of the conduct in question. When I asked a senior official of the HPC why the medical profession has no code of ethics, I was informed, 'what we have in our booklet is only a guideline and individual professions are expected to draw their own, but we can not say you must'. The British counterpart of the HPC, the GMC, has got the famous Blue Book, *Professional Conduct and Discipline: Fitness to Practise*, which formally outlines standards of professional conduct, medical ethics, kinds of misconduct that may invoke disciplinary action and the general disciplinary processes.

The BMA has its own code of ethics, *The Handbook of Medical Ethics*, unlike its Zimbabwean counterpart, the ZMA, which does not. In an interview, one senior ZMA official informed me that everyone knows the Hippocratic Oath and therefore there was no need to have a code, and that in any case the general code of ethics drawn by the Council is adequate. It is quite possible that the ZMA has deliberately decided to do without because lack of a code protects individual doctors, even though this taints its professional image as a whole. The picture of medical practise unfolding in Zimbabwe seems to confirm Johnson's (1973) argument that the practise of an occupation in a different context does not automatically imbue that profession with the professional qualities that it is associated with in another context. The situation of the Zimbabwean medical profession is even worse than Johnson envisaged, as parents of one malpractice victim remarked, 'we have been shocked to discover the extent to which medicine [in Zimbabwe] ... seems to be operating in an ethical vacuum' (Rothman and Rothman, 22 October, 1992:22).

The University of Zimbabwe medical school curriculum had almost no input on medical ethics until the curriculum was reviewed in 1994 (Medical School Curriculum Review, 1992). Given this, it is not surprising that the profession could again not agree on the ethicality of the 1994 doctors' strike. Almost all the junior doctors felt that striking was ethically acceptable, as one of them put it, 'ethics are a grey area and vary from person to person', while some consultants and expatriate doctors felt that it the strike was not ethically acceptable. What is ethically acceptable to a group should be known to all members of that group, especially in contexts where the group has the right to regulate itself and where discretionary decisions made in the course of its duties can have grave consequences for clients. The medical profession was granted the right to be tried by its own standards, but is unable to state what those standards are in the Zimbabwean context. The ignorance of self-regulation and the implicit social contract among Zimbabwean doctors was illustrated by one consultant who asked me, 'why should society expect doctors and lawyers to behave ethically when everyone else is doing what they want ... what is this calling?'

How Disciplinary Cases Come to the HPC

According to the Medical, Dental and Allied Professions Act (chapter 224) allegations against practitioners can come from members of the public, employers or other registered persons. In addition, the courts are supposed to pass on to the HPC criminal cases concerning persons registered with that body. One of the main problems is that most members of the public do not know of the existence of the HPC, its functions, the kinds of behaviour that constitute misconduct, and procedures for lodging a complaint. There is nothing written to inform the public of its existence and how complaints are lodged with it. In the course of the interviews, it became clear that even some consultants are not quite clear about the regulatory role of the Council and what this actually entails. One consultant asked me in interviews why the HPC behaves like the police force instead of protecting the medical doctors in what she deemed to be the manner of the BMA.

In the absence of an ethical code most members of the public do not know the kinds of offences for which they can complain to the HPC and in any case, most are not able to tell whether or not the doctor's behaviour is responsible for the negative outcome. The information gap between most members of the public and medical practitioners makes it rare for aggrieved members of the public to lodge a complaint. Inability to detect malpractice is common in most countries, regardless of the socio-economic status of the patient. Apparently, some mistakes can only be detected by peers and, even then, there is disagreement except for the very grossest of mistakes (Rosenthal, 1995). Even when the mistakes are quite obvious, most patients are extremely reluctant to complain, as one British health manager remarked to Rosenthal, 'it never ceases to amaze me how few complaints we get about the one we know is incompetent. People are so resistant to complaining. Why don't people complain? Is there no faith in the system? Are their expectations so low' (Rosenthal, 1995:26)?

In more or less the same vein, one consultant informed me in an interview that sometimes he advises his patients to sue him because of a bad surgical outcome, but they will not do so. The majority of Zimbabweans do not lodge complaints for cultural and financial reasons and also because there are no precedents of successful malpractice cases in the country, as discussed below. Revelations of the Parliamentary Select Committee investigating the HPC showed that there is considerable evidence of malpractice ending in loss of life, yet only one medical practitioner has been struck off the register since independence. If Rosenthal's (1995) estimates that at least 5 per cent of all licensed physicians in the United States and other countries are either incompetent or unscrupulous is anything to go by, there are many cases going undetected in Zimbabwe. The public is almost totally unprotected by the HPC, which does not have its own investigative structure, such as an inspectorate for uncovering professional and clinical offences by doctors and other professionals.

Health professionals are supposed to notify the HPC about misconduct by colleagues in accordance with Instrument 93 of 1993, but this is thwarted by their reluctance to report on each other, as discussed in Chapter 5. The Parliamentary Select Committee investigating the HPC found that some peri-operative deaths were not reported to the medical superintendent and to the police, even though this has always been mandatory. The small size of the medical population in the country makes it difficult for doctors to testify as expert witnesses in cases involving colleagues. In the United States, the informer laws made it mandatory for doctors to report on each other and the profession as a whole is beginning to take self-regulation more seriously in order to recover lost public trust (Freidson, 1989).

The case of Dr McGowan, which is discussed in full later, illustrates doctors' reluctance to report on each other. Even though he is a private anaesthetist, some of the deaths took place in Parirenyatwa hospital. In 1992, he anaesthetized a patient who died within twenty four hours of an operation at Parirenyatwa Hospital, carried out a post-mortem, even though a doctor is not supposed to carry out a post-mortem on a patient on whom he or she has worked, and had the body released and sent out of the country, and yet none of the health workers reported the case. In Britain, Rosenthal (1995) found that doctors find it extremely difficult to act against incompetent colleagues because of the cultural norm of turning away unless they have bad relations with them.

In the course of interviews, it emerged that some HPC officials know medical practitioners who settle cases out of court, yet no disciplinary measures are taken. Some HPC officials voiced their suspicion that some of the offending doctors were in fact advised by senior HPC officials to settle out of court in order to avoid disciplinary action. Out of court settlements mean that the practitioner is not disciplined and is also saved the public embarrassment and inconvenience of a court case. In addition, an out of court settlement is secretive, and colleagues do not get to know of the offence and cannot stop referring patients to the doctor, a commonly used mechanism for dealing with incompetent colleagues in other countries (Rosenthal, 1995). The financial cost to the doctor of out of court settlements are low and non-prohibitive in Zimbabwe and, in any case, these are paid for them by the Medical Defence Union, UK.

200

The screening body of the Council is supposed to be the Executive Committee comprising nine members, two of whom are medical practitioners, and chaired by the HPC President, a doctor. After receiving a complaint, the Executive Committee is supposed to ask the accused for a written representation, after which it carries out an initial investigation to determine whether the allegations constitute improper or disgraceful conduct, or gross incompetence. If the Executive Committee determines that the allegation is neither, the President may admonish the doctor, and report to Council, justifying the action taken, but if the Executive Committee considers the evidence adequate, the case is referred to the Disciplinary Committee for further investigation. The members of the Disciplinary Committee, which includes at least one non-medical HPC member, are appointed by the HPC President with the advice of the Executive Council and three people including the chairperson, form a quorum, with the latter given a deliberative as well as a casting vote. A legal member of the HPC is also supposed to be present to advise Council. While the defendant is allowed legal counsel the complainant is not. Once a decision has been made, the complainant has no right of appeal and if they are not satisfied with the verdict, the only recourse is to the courts.

The Disciplinary Committee is far too small to reflect a wide range of opinions and to allow for differences of opinion. It does not, like the British GMC and the Swedish MRB, include lay members, hence it is difficult for such a small group to disagree, especially where there are shared values between most of the members and the defendant. Indeed, it is quite possible that they will all know the defendant. In comparison, the Professional Conduct Committee of the GMC comprises twenty members and, even though the majority are medical professionals, the large size of the committee allows for differences of opinion. The Swedish MRB, comprising nine members, is smaller than the British Professional Conduct Committee, but makes up for this by having other professionals and lay people who can be objective.

Once the Disciplinary Committee has made a decision, the matter is reported to the Council, which will direct the registrar to implement sanctions. The type of sanctions at the disposal of the Disciplinary Committee include: removal from the register or suspension from practising for a specified period; imposition of conditions on the practising certificate; payment of a fine not exceeding Z$1,000 (less than 100 pounds sterling) to the Council; payment of any costs arising from the inquiry; censure; caution; or no further action. Any person aggrieved by the sanctions imposed can appeal to the High Court within three months of the decision being made.

In practise, however, the Registrar, a lay person (the current one is a former police officer) of the HPC single-handedly screens the letters of complaints and writes to the complainant asking for more details and then decides whether the case needs further investigation or not. This is largely because the Executive Committee does not meet often enough to act as a screening committee and therefore tends to rely heavily on the administrative staff. In interviews, the Registrar stated that most of the cases do not go further because they are due to breakdown in communication between the doctor and his or her client. A copy of the complaint is sent to the doctor for his or her response and, if it appears to the Registrar that there is a case to answer, the doctor is advised accordingly and the case is referred to the Disciplinary Committee.

There is much more reliance on lay administrative staff in Zimbabwe than, for example, in the Swedish context, yet their suitability for that role has not been an issue. Members of the Council who were interviewed explained that when the Council meets, there are so many issues to consider that they are not able to give much attention to individual disciplinary cases which means that, in effect, decisions on whether there was improper or disgraceful conduct or gross incompetence are made by the Registrar and his administrative staff during the preliminary screening. One member of the Council interviewed by the Parliamentary Select Committee investigating the HPC stated that in a year the Disciplinary Committee only dealt with three cases, the rest having been disposed of by the Registrar and his administrative team (Parliamentary Select Committee Report, 1993). This resembles the GMC where the chairperson and his administrative staff carry out the preliminary screening and dispose of up to 75 per cent of the cases (Robinson, 1989). In Sweden, on the other hand, a judge, who is the chairperson of the MRB, only disposes 6 per cent of the cases on his own and the rest are considered by the whole MRB after investigation by the 50 professional health staff whose duty is to investigate cases involving members of their own profession. This raises the issue of their competence and qualifications to carry out such a task since none have a background in health care at all and it is unlikely that they can effectively determine improper or disgraceful conduct or gross negligence in the absence of profession-specific codes of conduct. The ideal situation would be to have lay persons and professionals in both the screening committee and the disciplinary committee, rather than the current situation, where screening is done entirely by lay persons and decision-making in the disciplinary committee is done almost entirely by members of the defendant's profession.

It is paradoxical that the Zimbabwean doctors maintain that other health workers and lay persons cannot understand the technical aspects of medicine and therefore cannot effectively participate in their regulation, yet in fact, most of the cases, are determined by even less qualified persons. Robinson (1989) argues that informed lay people listen to the evidence and try to reach an honest verdict and if there is a code of conduct, even a lay person would be able to know when there has been a deviation from the code by the defendant.

In the Swedish system, all cases are considered and investigated but the sentences are generally light, although a practising certificate can be withdrawn for giving insufficient information about diagnosis, risks, complications, erroneous diagnosis and other technical errors (Rosenthal, 1987). The GMC, on the other hand, is supposed to be concerned with serious issues at the expense of less serious ones and negligence cases, but disciplinary action on those judged to be guilty of serious professional misconduct is very heavy (Rosenthal, 1987; Stacey, 1992). The Zimbabwean system combines the weaknesses of the Swedish and the British systems in considering only serious misconduct and giving light sentences. For example, in 1982, a senior surgeon took a patient from a government hospital and let his nine year old step son amputate a leg while he took a video of it which was shown on an American television programme. The Disciplinary Committee fined him Z$500 and that was the end of it. It was only due to public outcry that the Government banned him from its hospitals and he subsequently left for South Africa. Not surprisingly the Parliamentary Select Committee (1992 :12) concluded that, 'both within and outside the medical profession there exists a widespread belief grounded on experience that Council exists in order to cover up for bad doctors and not in order to promote justice and good medicine'.

In the past, the proceedings of the Council were regularly reported in the local medical journal, the *Central African Medical Journal (CAJM)*, but this was discontinued in 1985 with the change of the editorial team of the journal. On inquiring why this practice was stopped, I was informed by an HPC official that it was not in the interest of the Council and that 'people are not interested in everyday staff. Proceedings of the Council are private and confidential'. If the Council is there to protect the public, why should the public be denied access to such vital information which helps them in their choice of doctor and hospital?

Other Regulatory Mechanisms

Law courts/litigation The purposes of the legal system in medical regulation are to identify possible malpractice; provide compensation; and deter future negligence. On its own it is an inadequate regulatory system because, in any society, the ability and inclination to sue is not an option which is equally accessible to everyone (Klein, cited in Foreword in Rosenthal, 1987). Its utilisation and effectiveness as a regulatory mechanism is influenced by a number of factors, ranging from the cultural, socio-economic and political tradition of the society, the effectiveness of the police in building a case, the compensatory system, and the commitment and diligence of the prosecution.

In Zimbabwe, the police has the duty to establish the possibility of malpractice or liability and to initiate prosecutions against doctors in cases of peri-operative or maternal deaths. They also play a preliminary, but central role, in the investigations where complainants want to sue, hence, the effectiveness of the court system as a regulatory measure depends heavily on the skill and effectiveness of the police in collecting the evidence on which the prosecution depends. The legal system can only work as a regulatory mechanism if it is utilised by aggrieved patients and relatives suing medical practitioners if they are unhappy with the process or outcome of treatment. In Zimbabwe, rarely are cases brought to court for wrong diagnosis, inadequate information or technical errors, other than for surgical instruments left inside patients following surgical operations. The lack of information for patients and their relatives has limited the cases brought to court to those classified as peri-operative which can easily be linked to medical intervention.

All peri-operative deaths are supposed to be reported to the police who should investigate the circumstances of the death and prepare a docket for the case to be submitted to the Attorney General's Office. The Parliamentary Select Committee found that the police was often not informed of some peri-operative deaths and could therefore not investigate them (Parliamentary Select Committee, 1993). Moreover, police investigations largely depend on autopsy reports provided by government pathologists but some magistrates complained about the uninformative nature of the autopsy reports provided (Parliamentary Select Committee, 1993). The Committee found, after interviewing the police, that most did not know why they carried out the procedures which are central to the building of a case for prosecution. For that reason, some important information was not provided because the police did not understand its significance and therefore were not able to ask for clearer and more informative reports from the pathologists. Not surprisingly, opportunities of pursuing cases of possible malpractice were often lost. The Committee also found that the doctors' reports often gave uninformative causes of death and used medical jargon which the police often could not comprehend. For example, death certificates could state that a patient had died of apnoea (stopped breathing) or cardiac arrest, without stating the underlying cause. The committee also found that the education and social gap between the medical profession and the police made the latter timid to interrogate doctors.

University and government consultants interviewed stated that most of the doctors who work as pathologists in government hospitals are 'half-baked and do not know what they are talking about'. In addition, police officers who would like to do their job diligently sometimes run into professional problems, for example, the police officer who investigated the McGowan case faced harassment from the business sector, the legal and medical professions, the police and the Attorney General's Office and he was eventually transferred to a less desirable station (*ZimRights News*, December 1993).

The effectiveness of the police is only one step in a long legal process. Whether the case stands a chance in succeeding or not also depends on the diligence and commitment of the Attorney General's Office. The Parliamentary Select Committee found that as many as twenty one dockets on medical offences were closed prematurely without adequate investigation and that the Attorney General's Office was generally hostile to plaintiffs. Dr McGowan was only indicted two and half years after the case was first reported and largely due to public and international pressure (*ZimRights News*, December 1993).

Some patients and relatives may have doubts or be unhappy about the doctors' conduct or the outcome of a treatment, but they are highly unlikely to complain. Hill (1987) quotes the Medical Defense Union as saying that Zimbabweans hardly ever sue, 'patients are grateful for the medical attention received and in any case are not litigious' (Rothman and Rothman, 22 October, 1992). The President of the ZMA and the lawyer representing the Medical Defence Union (MDU) in Zimbabwe informed me that contributions to the MDU have more than trebled in the last five years, partly because of increased claims, but the lawyer could not say more because the information is confidential.

Prohibitively high legal fees are another important reason for lack of legal action by Zimbabwean patients and relatives. It is illegal for Zimbabwean lawyers to accept a case on a contingency fee as happens in the United States. Complainants who win their lawsuit are awarded damages only for lost income and out of pocket expenses and not for pain and suffering. In the case of a child, damages are limited to medical and funeral costs and this would be less than the lawyers' fees (Rothman and Rothman, 1992:23). Moreover, there is a shortage of lawyers with skills relevant to successfully pursuing medical malpractice cases and, consequently, the success rate is low and this discourages others from suing.

According to Zimbabwean law, an employer is liable for employee's acts committed in the course of carrying out their duties (Feltoe and Nyapadi,1989). While, this law does not exempt practitioners from liability for their actions, Feltoe and Nyapadi point out that a decision to sue the hospital only is often taken because it is thought that it is in a better position to pay substantial damages. The legal system is therefore not an effective regulatory mechanism with regards to government-employed doctors something of which they themselves are aware of.

Medical professional associations Associations are supposed to set the minimum standard of behaviour expected of members, with a code of conduct or ethics. In the United States, the American Medical Association (AMA) does promote high standards of practise by its members and other interests in the health sector by setting minimum standards of health services for drug manufacturers, dietary foods, therapeutic and diagnostic services (Freidson, 1988). It promotes high standards among its members by giving research awards; and promotes communication of scientific knowledge and procedures through its journals, lecture programmes and conventions (Freidson, 1988). Professional association membership is important for a doctor's career in the United States since it is difficult to get appointed to the staff of a hospital without this. In addition, there is a higher insurance premium for those who are not members, indeed sometimes insurance cover can even be denied. The AMA is, therefore, perceived as an effective regulator and membership is attractive to doctors because of the opportunities it affords.

As pointed out in Chapter 4, the main attraction of ZMA is that it has managed to negotiate lower membership rates with the Medical Defence

Union. Other than that, there does not seem to be any other attraction or benefit, except for the executive members who may be appointed to some boards under the Ministry of Health. It does not give research awards, it does not have a journal of its own nor does it provide continuing education for its members and there are no employers who require ZMA membership. In fact, it does not even provide legal aid for its members, as happens with the Swedish Medical Association and has not especially portrayed itself as an organisation that promotes the financial interests of its members. As we noted earlier, it was precisely because of this lack of support for hospital-based doctors that the latter decided to form the HDA. Membership of ZMA is not beneficial and denying anyone membership as a sanction is not effective because one does not lose much.

The ZMA does not have a code of ethics and has not set a minimum standard of practice and competence for its members, which means that it is not even trying to convince an anxious public that it promotes good medicine. While its officials were horrified by the methods used by Dr McGowan and asked the Council to look at them as far back as 1986, it only reacted in the wake of public outcry over the case in 1993 (Parliamentary Select Committee, 1993). The then president of ZMA wrote to the Minister of Health asking him to consider the possibility of introducing medical audit in various institutions in view of an 'adverse media campaign against the profession' (Mundawarara, quoted in the Parliamentary Select Committee, 1993:21). This casts doubt on the sincerity of the organisation to improve performance, as its emphasis seems to be on staving off political interference. The ZMA has also made efforts to improve its public image by suggesting a patients' rights charter, but it all appears to be a public relations exercise rather than genuine desire to protect the interests of the public. From the above evidence, we can conclude that the ZMA has no effective regulatory function on its members.

As pointed out above, the College of Primary Care Physicians is an organisation of general practitioners, with membership largely limited to white and older black doctors. Of the three existing organisations, it is the only one which offers continuing education. Its failure to secure HPC's recognition of its proposed examinations as a requisite for entry into private practice deprived it of a useful weapon.

It is, however, the only association which has pointed out the need for more effective medical regulation for both government-employed and private doctors (CPCP, 1992). It suggested the establishment of disciplinary and ethical committees within the professional bodies, and the passing of information on unethical colleagues. The patients consulting its members have minimum protection, given that doctors do not work in a medical firm structure where other doctors are likely to pick out mistakes made by a colleague. In spite of its apparent concern with patient welfare, its effectiveness has been significantly reduced by its internal and racial divisions, as manifested in its lack of public response in both the 1994 doctor's strike and the McGowan case discussed above.

The HDA is primarily concerned with improving the economic and working conditions of its members. The membership is voluntary, and the HDA executive admitted that a considerable number have not paid their membership fees although they benefit from the organisation's trade union activities. The organisation has not wanted to alienate its members by pushing the issue of membership fees because it benefits by having everyone supporting it during strike action. It has no sanctions at its disposal than other the disapproval of other members.

The organisation has not been especially concerned about the welfare of patients. It has not said anything about its members practising privately when their certificates do not allow this. In conclusion, one can argue that the HDA has fought very effectively for the interests of its members, but not for the regulation of their performance or level of competence and public accountability.

Consumer/patient and civil action In the British context, patients' associations and victims' organisations have made a tremendous contribution in strengthening regulation of the medical profession by the GMC (Robinson, 1989; Stacey, 1992). In the Zimbabwean context, there are no civil organisations specifically concerned with patients' problems or with victims of malpractice, such as the Victims of Medical Accidents in Britain, and aggrieved patients and relatives have not attempted to work as a group to pursue justice from the medical profession or health institutions. The struggle for economic survival which is the primary concern of the majority of the population, means that access to health care is the issue rather than the quality of that care.

The Consumer Council of Zimbabwe stated that it has no capacity to deal with cases of medical malpractice. A number of human rights organisations have taken up the case of patients after they have failed to get a response through the normal channels, but this is a very recent development which occurred in the wake of the McGowan case. Unfortunately, the organisations have no sanctions at their disposal other than bad publicity for the individual or institution concerned. *ZimRights News* and some privately owned newspapers have enabled some aggrieved people to air their grievances against the medical profession and the health sector in general. People who have tried to obtain justice through the normal channels have been able to tell their stories to the newspapers and some are suing the doctors almost ten years later (*Horizon*, June 1995).

The regulatory role of Parliament   The Ministry of Health is ultimately answerable to parliament, as a government department and periodically, parliamentary committees examine the operations of government service ministries and report their findings. For example, the 1992/93 report expressed severe disquiet at the abuse of government hospital beds by private doctors and the breakdown and shortage of equipment at Parirenyatwa and other hospitals. These Committees can force ministry officials to examine the issues raised and their findings can be publicised by the newspapers. Members of Parliament can also ask the Ministry of Health to inform Parliament on the action that it has taken on certain issues raised by Parliamentary Committees. Their role is useful, but the Minister can oppose or ignore their demands, as happened when some called for an investigation into the McGowan case.

Another parliamentary regulatory mechanism employed in Zimbabwe is that of the Comptroller and Auditor General's Office. His investigation of the central hospitals, including Parirenyatwa, revealed the frequent absence from government hospitals of consultants employed there and the reluctance of the Ministry of Health officials to discipline them. The report can generate interest when picked up by the media but otherwise its findings go largely unnoticed by the public.

Parliament can also set up special committees to look at the role and operations of particular institutions, as happened in 1992 with investigations into the functions of the HPC. As a response, the ZMA advised its members to establish medical audit and the Ministry of Health passed Statutory Instrument 93 of 1993 and started restructuring the HPC. There were, however, many other recommendations made by the Committee which the Ministry of Health has not implemented, which seems to point to the limited role of parliament as a regulatory mechanism. The ability and effectiveness of parliament on regulating government departments depends on their responsiveness to its authority but the real power lies with the state President who appoints the ministers.

The McGowan case illustrates how the entire medical disciplinary machinery works, particularly its deficiencies. As pointed out earlier, this case made the issue of medical discipline topical in the country when the parents of a victim who died at the hands of Dr McGowan exhausted the whole disciplinary machinery in a bid to have justice carried out. This particular case took place in a private hospital but the doctor also had operating rights in Parirenyatwa Hospital.

In August 1990, a ten year old black Kenyan girl died in Zimbabwe where her father, a lawyer, was based. The child had been admitted to Avenues Clinic, the biggest private hospital in Harare, for an appendicectomy. The parents talked to their child after the operation and then left after the visiting hour in the evening. At 2100 hours that same evening they were summoned by the hospital and informed that the child had collapsed, but when they arrived at the hospital she was already dead. They sought audience with the anaesthetist, who only told them that the child had suddenly stopped breathing and the surgeon who had operated was not able to offer an explanation at all.

The parents asked the Chief Executive Officer of Avenues Clinic to provide details of the incident and to order an investigation, but he refused to do so on the pretext that the hospital was not legally responsible for the activities of the practitioners who use its facilities and arguing that 'all the patients are admitted in the care of their medical practitioners. The facilities, equipment and nursing care only are provided by the clinic' (Rothman and Rothman, 1992:22).

The parents managed, with much difficulty, to secure their child's hospital chart and to have three doctors of their choice present when the autopsy was carried out. The autopsy revealed that the anaesthetic method employed was not commonly used and that the child had not received adequate post-operative care. The parents took the evidence to the HPC, which agreed to investigate the case but did not ask them to submit the autopsy reports which they had. They were not permitted to hear or review the evidence submitted by others on the case, and when they asked about the progress of the case after three months, they were informed that 'it is not Council policy to apprise a complainant of the procedures adopted and to issue progress reports. When the investigation is completed, you will be advised' (Rothman and Rothman, 1992:21).

After several more inquiries without success, the parents were able to secure audience with the head of the Council who immediately handed them a letter before talking to them. The letter stated,

> The Council has now completed its investigation ... and determined there was no negligence or incompetence on the part of the surgeon, the anaesthetist or the nursing staff at the ... clinic. The anaesthetist followed recognised procedures and the nursing staff carried out their duties in accordance with the doctor's (written) instructions. (Rothman and Rothman, 1992:22)

As far as the Council was concerned, the case was closed, but the dissatisfied parents lobbied the medical associations to investigate the case, without success. But, fortunately for the parents, because this was peri-operative death, the police was obliged to investigate. After the autopsy findings already referred to were released to them, the police concluded that there was a case to be answered as a matter of urgency, but their inquiries took a very long time. When the parents asked the Attorney General's office for progress of the case, they were told to exercise restraint. To strengthen their case, they investigated other incidents involving the same anaesthetist and found several others, including one of death during an operation to remove gall stones, a case of brain damage following circumcision, and a death following a tooth extraction.

Two months after the death of their child, the parents, frustrated from lack of action by the police and the Council, appealed to university students and the most well known human rights organisation in the country, the Catholic Commission for Justice and Peace. The students and the Commission organised a demonstration and marched towards the hospital where the child had died and to the offices of the HPC. Some members of parliament introduced a resolution asking for a public inquiry into allegations of malpractice at the private hospital, but the Minister of Health, Dr Stamps, gave an impassioned speech in defence of the medical profession and the hospital, which he said was providing high cost care at no cost to the tax payer. The Minister further argued that an inquiry would be contrary to the interests of the country. He insisted that the anaesthetic method employed on the child was 'conventional, safe and time honoured ... widely used world wide in many tertiary units ... open heart surgery would be impossible without this procedure' (*Parliamentary Debates*, 21 November, 1990). The Minister also castigated press coverage of the case, which he described as 'inappropriate and unacceptable ... not consistent with good public order' (*Parliamentary Debates*, 21 November, 1990). The impact of the Minister's performance in parliament was that an inquiry was staved off for one and half years.

In desperation, the parents decided to appeal to Africa Watch, a New York based international organisation which documents and publicises human rights abuses in Africa. They wrote asking for help 'to enable us to continue our legal struggle to bring to book those responsible for the death of our child' (Rothman and Rothman, 1992:21). The organisation sent two people to investigate the case and the published report elicited a lot of interest, both locally and internationally and after this, Parliament adopted a motion appointing a select committee to investigate the functioning of the HPC on 19 March, 1992.

When the Parliamentary Select Committee report was released there was a public outcry. It showed that the first death had occurred in 1986 after the use of the same procedure by Dr McGowan and the Parliamentary Select Committee identified five deaths which had occurred after the use of the procedure. The report alleged that he was involved in clinical trials and he personally admitted to being involved in attempts to 'break new ground in medical techniques' (*Parliamentary Debates*, 4 March, 1993). He admitted that he had initiated the trials without obtaining the necessary permission from the Drugs Control Council, the Secretary for Health or from the patients and their relatives before carrying out the procedure, as laid down by the Drugs Control Act of 1987. The anaesthetist was charged with five counts of murder arising from his unauthorised medical experiments, thirty months after the case was first reported to the police.

The revelation by the Parliamentary Select Committee that a lot of health workers, institutions and organisations had misgivings about the anaesthetist's method and its effect on patients and yet had done nothing was dubbed a 'conspiracy of silence'. The Ministry of Health quickly drafted Statutory Instrument 93 of 1993 with the aim of forcing health workers and institutions to report behaviour that has a negative impact on the welfare of patients.

In September 1993, the Council, which had earlier fully absolved Dr McGowan of any wrong doing, issued him a restrictive practising certificate which prohibited him from using the offending anaesthetic method in operations, but he contravened the conditions endorsed on his certificate and used the method again at Avenues Clinic. A nurse reported the case to the authorities and he was barred from practising in that hospital and also from St Annes Hospital. He had already been banned from the Parirenyatwa

Group of Hospitals in 1992. When the HPC informed the anaesthetist of its intention to discipline him for contravening the restrictions on his certificate, he appealed to the High Court and an order was granted barring the Council from convening a disciplinary hearing until the court case was concluded. His argument was that 'many medical practitioners have sworn affidavits to the effect that it is not in the public interest for me to be barred from performing epidural anaesthesia' (*Daily Gazette*, 13 January, 1994). The high court lifted the conditions imposed on his license on the pretext that he needed the money from practising medicine to meet his legal costs.

There were protests by human rights groups and university students, some of whom went on hunger strike in protest to the British government, which had allegedly sent the Princess of Wales to ask the Zimbabwean government to lift the conditions imposed on his practising licence by the Health Professions Council. This did not achieve anything except to highlight the public's suspicion of the perceived injustice of the High Court decision. The British High Commission explained that the Princess of Wales, who had visited the country on behalf of the Red Cross, had nothing to do with the court decision and that the case was not even discussed in her meeting with the state President. Whatever the merits of the story, it graphically portrays the Zimbabwe public's perception of the justice system, the role of the state in the judiciary system and the amenability of the state to the influence of foreign powers and institutions.

After a long protracted process, the anaesthetist, who had initially been charged with five counts of murder, later reduced to culpable homicide, was in January 1995 convicted on two counts of medical negligence both resulting in the death of patients. He was sentenced to six months imprisonment by a black judge and refused bail but, a white chief justice overruled him the very next day and granted bail pending an appeal and also allowed him to practise while awaiting appeal. The verdict was received with disbelief and anger by the parents and relatives of the victims, the human rights organisations and the majority of the black population. In the minds of many, it just confirmed what they had long suspected, that justice would not be realised because of the race of the accused, connections with powerful people and government's fear of alienating international donors.

The above case further highlights the perfunctory manner in which complaints are often dealt with by the Council. There were several deaths linked to the doctor reported to the Council, and yet no serious investigation was carried out. The inconsistency of the Council became apparent when,

213

after stating that Dr McGowan's method was acceptable, it later imposed conditions on his practising certificate. The absence of regulation of private health institutions and the lack of protection of patients in those institutions which the Ministry of Health had sought to remedy with the Health Services and Institutions Bill were highlighted. It was revealed by the Parliamentary Select Committee, no one is responsible for the clinical performance of medical doctors at Avenues Clinic, as the Chief Executive is a pharmacist by training.

Most of the deaths that were revealed by the Parliamentary Select Committee took place at Avenues Clinic, which is not necessarily a reflection of a high level of negligence on the part of the staff, but of the middle class who go there. One other issue which arose was that doctors in this hospital, as in other private clinics, write very little notes on the patient as a protective mechanism. The Chief Executive of the Avenues Clinic informed in interview that some reorganisation was undertaken to rectify some of the shortcomings pointed out by the Parliamentary Select Committee.

Conclusions

The aim of this chapter has been to analyze the regulation of medical education, registration and discipline and the nature and extent of autonomy which the medical profession exercises in this respect. We noted that a number of institutions are involved in regulating these aspects but that the HPC is the body ultimately responsible for medical regulation. Although the HPC is answerable to government, in practise the people who make the decisions are medical professionals in decision-making positions in various regulatory institutions and in the HPC itself.

Medical professionals in the medical school determine the entry qualifications into the medical school although the state has a final say by virtue of its control of the finances. With regards to the curriculum, the needs of the government are taken into account as much as possible but as the decision-makers are doctors themselves, they attempt as much as possible to ensure that it is internationally acceptable to facilitate employment and post-graduate education in developed countries. The study revealed that medical education, particularly internship and post-graduate education, is inadequately regulated by the doctors in decision-making positions in the responsible organisations who are currently benefitting from the *status quo*. Although the HPC effectively regulates the registration of locally trained doctors through its Practise Control Committee, it has however, failed to devise effective means to ensure that doctors registered with it retain their professional competence.

After examining the available evidence we must conclude that government-employed doctors are not effectively monitored and disciplined by the various regulatory structures. The definition of acts of misconduct outlined by the Public Service Disciplinary Regulations (1992), the main mechanism for regulating government-employed doctors, is inadequate for addressing medical offences and the sanctions proposed are equally irrelevant to the nature of those offences. The regulatory procedures are not only cumbersome and time consuming, but their effectiveness is further compromised by the inadequacy of the monitoring mechanisms. Before regulatory procedures can be initiated, those charged with that task need to be aware that an offence has occurred. The findings of this thesis show that the medical firm structure which is supposed to provide an in-built supervisory role is not working efficiently at the Parirenyatwa Group of Hospitals because of a shortage of registrars but also because some consultants spend more time in their private offices leaving their juniors without supervision. The performance reports which could be both a deterrent and a sanction for junior and middle rank doctors have been rendered ineffective by some consultants who indiscriminately give good reports. The adamant refusal by almost all the doctors to report on each other in accordance with the provisions of Instrument 93, further ensures that the medical superintendent who is supposed to initiate the disciplinary procedures is unaware of some of the medical offences. The channels through which patients could lodge their complaints against health personnel were not clearly articulated until 1995, when the first public relations officer was appointed. But unfortunately, offences coming through the public relations officer also have to be addressed through the cumbersome and ineffective Public Service disciplinary machinery. In addition to the ineffectiveness of the disciplinary machinery itself, it has also been revealed that there is a general reluctance to discipline doctors even when their offences are detected and reported.

Government-employed doctors who treat the majority of patients are almost unregulated by the HPC because of poor coordination between it and the Public Service regulatory structures. The HPC, on the other hand, has proved quite ineffective as a body responsible for regulating the medical profession because of a high threshold of what constitutes medical offences, the inefficient screening process, the domination of the HPC by the medical profession, and the small size of the disciplinary committee. The lack of an inspectorate to detect offences severely reduces the number of offences brought before the HPC particularly as the majority of people are unaware of its existence and can therefore not lodge complaints with the HPC. The ineffectiveness of the HPC as a regulatory structure is further compounded by the fact that the sanctions that it imposes are almost consistently too light to act as an effective deterrent.

Almost all the other institutions responsible for regulating medical discipline are equally ineffective. The effectiveness of the law courts depends on people's willingness to use them, the effectiveness of the police, the pathologists and the prosecutors in building a strong case. The cultural beliefs of the majority of the population, their inability to judge medical treatment and its outcomes, the prohibitive legal costs, lack of expert malpractice lawyers, and the lack of meaningful financial redress for the aggrieved, have ruled out litigation as viable option for most Zimbabweans.

The medical associations in Zimbabwe have not been concerned with the maintenance of medical discipline and lack both the regulatory mechanisms and sanctions. The role of Parliament in medical regulation has been weakened by its lack of sanctions to force government departments to implement its recommendations. The activities of civil and consumer organisations have to date been sporadic, marginal and negligible.

8 Summary and Conclusions

Introduction

The main aim of this book has been to analyze the nature of professional autonomy exercised by government-employed doctors in Zimbabwe. Medical autonomy was analyzed in three major dimensions, that is: clinical autonomy; economic autonomy; and self-regulation of medical education, registration and discipline. The aim of this chapter is, first of all, to summarise the main findings of the book, highlighting the nature of the individual dimensions of medical autonomy in Zimbabwe. The second aim is to draw conclusions regarding the validity of current theoretical conceptualizations of medical autonomy in the Zimbabwean context, particularly Freidson's (1988) theory of medical dominance, deprofessionalisation as well as proletarianisation hypotheses which are currently prominent in theories of professional power in the West, and Johnson's model of the medical profession in colonial and post-colonial states in Africa. The third and final aim is to propose a model of medical autonomy in post-colonial states in Africa. As noted in Chapter 1, our knowledge of professional autonomy is based almost exclusively on work done in developed western countries and, consequently, we know very little about the contemporary situation in post-colonial and developing countries. The proposed model which grows out of the book represents a theoretical contribution and suggests new analytical tools that should be used in addition to those which currently exist in further research, particularly within developing countries.

Summary of Findings

In Chapter 3 we saw that the medical profession was an important group in Rhodesian colonial society which played a vital role in the colonisation, establishment and maintenance of Southern Rhodesia as a white settler state, as successive colonial governments attempted to create an environment for settlers comparable to, if not better than, that in Britain. As part of that general aim, the state endeavoured to ensure that medical practice and health

217

care provision in the colony were attractive for settlers and doctors. This gave the medical profession considerable influence in negotiations with the state over their conditions of service and in the determination of colonial health policy by virtue of its expertise, through the activities of its professional association (the BMA and later the RMA), the activities of physicians in administrative positions, and because of shared social, economic and political values with the ruling elite.

The state sheltered the white settler medical profession from economic hardship by granting it retainer fees when private practice was not lucrative enough for it to survive; removing competition from doctors trained in America and continental Europe by refusing to recognise their medical qualifications for a long time; further reducing competition by denying blacks access to medical training; giving doctors unlimited access to government hospitals and keeping hospital fees sub-economic, thus making private medicine affordable to more people; rejecting the recommendation by the Saints Commission to establish a national health service; making health insurance tax-free; and by the passing of the 1979 Medical Act which expanded the private medical market and ensured that the vocal urban black elite was reliant on the private health sector. The net effect of these government policies was to make the private medical sector lucrative and strong enough to stave off threats to its survival by the post-colonial government.

On assuming power in 1980, the post-colonial government proposed a number of heath policies intended to contribute towards the establishment of a racially desegregated, egalitarian and socialist society. Some of these policies, which included free health care, the legalisation of traditional medicine, a review of medical education, the introduction of a limited drug list, and the adoption of a bonding contract for Zimbabwe-trained medical graduates, had the potential to seriously hurt medical interests. Not surprisingly, some met with stiff resistance from the medical profession and other interested parties, which meant that they had to be either modified or reversed by the government. The junior doctors have used the strike weapon in order to force government to abandon or modify some of the policies (as we saw in Chapter 6), while middle level doctors resigned from government hospitals in large numbers for either the private medical sector or neighbouring countries. Their efforts in this respect were reinforced by the private economic sector, international finance institutions and donor countries which expressed their opposition to policies that had a negative impact on private medical practice. We noted in Chapters 1 and 4 that in

1991 the government was compelled to revise some of its earlier policies as a result of escalating fiscal constraints, culminating in the adoption of the IMF and World Bank-prescribed Economic Structural Adjustment Programme. The introduction of ESAP, as we saw in Chapters 5 and 6, resulted in an overall reduction of the health care budget, which in turn exacerbated the problem of serious shortages of equipment and drugs in the hospital, as will be recapped below.

Clinical Autonomy

We saw that all government-employed doctors have minimal administrative restrictions on the type and number of diagnostic tests and the type of treatment that they can carry out. Rather, their ability to carry out diagnostic tests and the treatments of their choice is determined by the availability of necessary equipment, the staff situation in the ward and in the relevant paramedical departments, and the socio-economic status of the patient in question. Doctors exercise a high degree of clinical autonomy in the treatment of Social Dimensions of Adjustment Fund (SDF) patients when the resources are available, and in the treatment of patients with health insurance who can afford to pay for the use of private diagnostic facilities and can procure drugs from private pharmacies when necessary. Treatment of cash-paying, low-income patients limits the doctors' clinical autonomy, as they have to be cost-conscious and sometimes settle for what they consider to be less efficacious alternatives in order to suit the patients' financial situation.

We noted that shortages of essential resources, breakdowns of equipment and staff problems in the paramedical departments either delay the production of diagnostic test results or produce sub-optimal ones. Similarly, shortages of nurses and other support staff inhibit doctors from prescribing necessary observations or other procedures for their patients. The shortage of doctors, particularly registrars, has left those at Parirenyatwa with a heavy workload and unable to practise medicine as they should. In spite of this, all grades of doctors have felt compelled to practise privately, sometimes during working hours, in order to supplement their government incomes, which they perceive as inadequate.

In Chapter 5 we noted that all grades of doctors exercise a considerable degree of autonomy in prescribing and consequently, that our assumption that Essential Drugs List of Zimbabwe (EDLIZ) would limit doctors' autonomy was not borne out by the findings of this thesis. Although doctors were not consulted when the policy was adopted, they were widely consulted in the drawing up of the drugs list. Unfortunately, although the EDLIZ has become progressively more comprehensive over the years, doctors are often unable to prescribe the drugs of their choice for SDF patients because, at any one time, some drugs are not available in the hospital pharmacy. Since the introduction of Economic Structural Adjustment Programme, however, doctors of all grades can prescribe drugs outside the list and patients can buy them from private pharmacies, but obviously this is only possible for those patients who can afford to buy them.

In the final analysis, we can conclude that all levels of doctors exercise more clinical autonomy than they would if the medical firm structure was functioning efficiently. Junior doctors, in particular, exercise more autonomy and carry out more serious medical and surgical procedures than they should at their level. Consultants also have more autonomy in the absence of effective medical audit systems and other mechanisms aimed at reviewing their clinical decisions, which increasingly impact on their counterparts in Britain and the United States. The autonomy of all grades of doctors has not yet been curtailed by controls prescribed by authoritative and prescriptive management intent on achieving quality and cost effectiveness.

While it would seem that doctors in the United States and increasingly in Britain (Summerton, 1995) are always conscious of the possibility of litigation for malpractice (Rosenthal, 1987), the majority of patients treated at Parirenyatwa Hospital are not aware of their rights and doctors take clinical decisions without much consideration of what, elsewhere, is perceived to be an external constraint. The greatest constraint on clinical autonomy confronting doctors at the Parirenyatwa Group of Hospitals stems from the overall shortage of resources in the hospitals. This is more severe than anything occurring in Britain and yet no serious and systematic attempt has been made to alter individual doctors' practising habits. So, instead of dealing with precisely planned managerial cost controls and constraints on autonomy like their counterparts in the United States, doctors at Parirenyatwa reduce each others' clinical autonomy through uncontrolled prescribing leading to shortage of drugs.

Economic Autonomy

In Chapter 6 we found that doctors working at Parirenyatwa Hospital exercise more economic autonomy than they should. Junior doctors have much more leverage than other health workers when negotiating their conditions of service, particularly as they have used the strike weapon effectively to push their demands with the government. The perennial shortage of doctors and the high turnover have made government indulgent in its regulation of doctors, leaving them with more autonomy than is desirable for good patient care. Doctors successfully challenged the bonding contract which was intended to give Government the right to determine how long they should work at designated institutions, including the less desirable rural hospitals, and to delay them from joining the private medical sector. Junior doctors led the protest which ended in the withdrawal of the Health Institutions and Services Bill (1989) which would have given government the right to determine the location of private health facilities and the conditions under which they operated. The medical profession's concerns about the likely impact of the Bill on private medicine were shared by the whole medical profession, but more importantly by the industrialists, who control the country's economy. The government, which was trying to entice foreign investors and donors, could not afford to ignore their voice.

At present the majority of junior doctors flagrantly contravene both the HPC regulations and government employment conditions by practising privately, with little regulation from the hospital management, the Ministry of Health, or the Health Professions Council, while middle level doctors who have not been able to obtain more favourable conditions of service in government have had the highest turnover from government institutions, forcing the government to rely on sometimes less suitable expatriate doctors. The terms of employment for government-employed consultants working at Parirenyatwa are comparable to those of their counterparts in the NHS and, as in Britain, most have been able to practise privately to a much greater extent than was intended in their imprecise contracts (Yates, 1995).

Government-employed consultants working at the Parirenyatwa Group of Hospitals have a right to attend an unspecified number of their own private patients in the hospital and are in fact, alleged to be spending more time with them than with SDF patients. In addition, government maintained, equipped and paid all paramedical staff at Mbuya Nehanda Maternity Hospital for use by government, university, and private consultants for 14 years and in return got sub-economic hospital fees, while consultants were privately and, no doubt handsomely, remunerated by their patients.

Our initial assumption that the introduction of free health care would erode doctors' economic autonomy was not confirmed. Free health care had no direct impact on the economic interests of government-employed doctors and, at most, a negligible one on the private medical sector, which is largely dependent on privately insured patients. Similarly, the legalisation of traditional medicine had no impact on the interests of government-employed doctors and their colleagues in private practice as the traditional practitioners cannot give certificates to their patients for official purposes, nor are they remunerated by health insurance organisations for their services. Consequently, the medical profession has retained its role as the gatekeeper to services in both government and private health institutions. It is highly unlikely that any of the services of traditional healers will ever be incorporated into government health institutions in the same manner that acupuncture and other alternative health practices are being incorporated in the NHS in Britain because the practitioners themselves fear such a move may enable the medical profession and the government to interfere in their clinical practices. But more importantly, government has not seriously expressed that intention.

From the above, we can say that all grades of doctors at Parirenyatwa exercise more economic autonomy than their counterparts in Britain, for example. On closer examination, however, it is evident that the basis of this autonomy is different from that exercised by counterparts in Britain and the United States which have stronger and more stable economies. Firstly, we noted that the Zimbabwe government's fiscal problems are relatively more severe and incapacitating than those experienced by Britain and the United States. Not only is the national economy declining, but so is the standard of living of the majority of the population, including medical professionals. Increasingly, most people are resorting to additional income generating activities to supplement their dwindling incomes. For doctors, as we noted, this has been in the form of private practice sometimes carried out during working hours. Senior management and administrators who find themselves in the same position have not done much to regulate such activities by their subordinates. Poor monitoring and reluctance to apply sanctions on recalcitrant doctors are relatively more prevalent in Zimbabwe than Britain, for example, where this behaviour is more common among consultants than other grades of doctors (Yates, 1995).

Regulation of Medical Education, Registration and Discipline

We noted in Chapter 7 that the Health Professions Council is dominated by the medical profession, as are its various committees which regulate medical education, registration and discipline. Even though the decisions made by the various HPC committees are ratified by a multi-professional HPC, they are rarely challenged.

In Chapter 7, we concluded that some aspects of medical education, such as internship and post-graduate education, are inadequately regulated. The HPC has not ordered an inspection of the medical school and teaching hospitals since independence in 1980, in spite of the doubling of the medical school intake twice in the last fifteen years, complaints about lack of supervision of interns, and excessive workloads which clearly contravene the terms initially set out when the medical school was opened; contravention of the terms of the internship by interns who are all practising privately; the introduction of many post-graduate medical programmes; and the high drop-out and failure rates of students registered on those programmes.

Although the HPC appears to do an adequate job when it comes to the registration of Zimbabwean doctors, it has not established a mechanism for ensuring that they retain their competence and for detecting those who have not. Similarly, it has not established a health committee to ensure that doctors or other health professionals who are ill are appropriately dealt with. Analysis of mechanisms for regulating medical discipline indicated that government employed-doctors are inadequately monitored and disciplined by the Public Service Disciplinary Procedures which are cumbersome and do not take into account the nature of clinical work and the potentially grave consequences of some medical offences.

The means for monitoring medical discipline in government hospitals are inefficient and, as result, most offences are not detected or reported. In addition, no effective channels have been established to enable the public to lodge their complaints. The proposed Patients' Rights Charter will inform patients on their rights and the channels for lodging complaints, but unfortunately, reported grievances will proceed through the cumbersome and fairly ineffective Public Service disciplinary procedures. No attempt has been made to coordinate the HPC and Public Service disciplinary structures to ensure that clinical offences committed by government-employed doctors are dealt with appropriately by the HPC. The net result of all these deficiencies is that government patients, who are supposed to be better protected than those treated in the private health sector, are, in fact, the most vulnerable because they are being treated by junior doctors with little supervision. The majority of patients treated at the Parirenyatwa Group of Hospitals tend to be less assertive and less inclined to complain or resort to litigation. Similarly, they are unlikely to exit from government hospitals because they cannot afford the services of private doctors.

The HPC itself has serious problems arising from the lack of ethical codes for the different health professions registered with it, even though its determination of what constitutes an offence is supposed to be based on ethical codes for each profession. The threshold of what constitutes medical misconduct is too high, and leaves some serious offences unregulated. In addition, the screening process is carried out by ill-qualified administrative staff because the relevant people are too busy. The inadequacies of the HPC are compounded by its lack of an inspectorate to detect offences, only reacting to those reported to it, but as we noted, the majority of ordinary people do not know of the existence of the HPC and how to lodge complaints with it. The small size of the Disciplinary Committee, its domination by the medical profession, and the whole disciplinary process tends to protect the doctor more than the complainant.

The other institutions responsible for regulating medical discipline, such as law courts, are also largely ineffective. Only a very small proportion of people resort to courts because they are often unable to determine when a malpractice has occurred, but also because of cultural and financial constraints. In any case, the success of law courts as a regulatory mechanism depends on the skill and commitment of police officers, pathologists, the Attorney General's Office and the prosecutors in collecting evidence and building a strong case. Unfortunately, the record to date is not encouraging and this makes the use of courts even less popular. The lack of meaningful compensation for victims of malpractice has further reduced the attractiveness of law courts as a medical regulatory mechanism.

Other regulatory mechanisms, such as Parliamentary Select Committees, Public Accounts Committees, and the Auditor and Comptroller General's reports, are effective at investigation and in publicising their findings, but have not always been able to force the Ministry of Health and Child Welfare to implement their recommendations. The professional associations have been altogether ineffective in regulating their members, and have in some instances adopted strategies to deflect more effective regulation by the government, as happened with the introduction of medical audit. There have not been any consumer groups or organisations concerned with patients, victims of medical malpractice or any issues to do with the quality of health care.

The above summary of medical autonomy in Zimbabwe suggests the situation differs somewhat from that in Britain and the United States on which most of the theories on professions have almost exclusively focused. The relevance of these theories in analysing the situation in developing countries forms the subject of the next section. Before assessing the relevance of each of these theories, it is necessary to very briefly restate their main propositions.

Assessing the Relevance of Current Theories of Professions

Dominance Theory

Firstly, Freidson (1988) asserts that medicine's status as an autonomous and most dominant occupation in the health care division of labour was legally conferred by the state, which continues to guarantee it. This special position was granted after the profession had convinced society, particularly the power elite, of its special skills, knowledge, trustworthiness and altruism. Secondly, Freidson states that medical associations lobbied government in order to secure professional status. Bjorkman (1989) argues that even in societies where the medical profession lacks an independent professional association, it can still wield considerable influence in state policy as a result of the activities of its members in decision-making positions in government.

Thirdly, in countering McKinlay and Arches' (1985) claims of proletarianisation, Freidson points out that employment status does not constitute the core element of professional dominance. Rather it is the value of goods and services to society that constitute the core and medicine continues to have high value, hence doctors continue to exercise control over the terms of their employment and content of their work (Freidson, 1989).

Fourthly, Freidson (1989) states that medical autonomy is under threat of erosion from authoritative management intent on achieving cost and quality control by introducing specific sets of procedures and protocols for judging doctors' work. He notes that this is increasingly taking control of medical work out of the hands of the rank and file into the hands of elite medical researchers and administrators. The ensuing stratification of the medical profession may be harmful to the internal cohesion of the corporate profession which is essential for the maintenance of its dominance. However, Freidson (1989) concludes that in spite of the changes in the nature of individual doctors' work, the medical profession as an entity retains its dominance because the responsibility of establishing clinical standards, reviewing performances and exercising supervision and control are carried out by members of the medical profession. In any case, the legal position of the medical profession has not changed and doctors have retained the sole authority to diagnose, treat, admit and discharge patients from hospitals.

With respect to the first point raised by Freidson, we found that the medical profession in Zimbabwe has dominance over other health workers not only at hospital level, but extending to all levels where policies on health care are formulated, including the positions of Minister of Health and Secretary for Health. We also noted that doctors at the Parirenyatwa Group of Hospitals exercise considerable clinical and economic autonomy, and the medical profession as an entity regulates medical education, licensing and discipline. But we noted that the medical profession in Zimbabwe did not emerge in the same manner that it did in Britain and the United States, as described by Freidson (1988) and Starr (1982). Rather, it was introduced into the colony along with other institutions during the colonial era, and inevitably, evolved differently because of the existing socio-economic and political conditions and the interrelationships among key forces comprising the state, other health care providers and the general public in the country. We noted that during the colonial era, the BMA and later the RMA were relatively strong and well organised and successfully lobbied the government whenever medical interests were threatened. Although the Zimbabwe Medical Association is weaker than its colonial predecessor, the medical profession continues to exercise autonomy in its work and to regulate medical education, licensing and discipline through the activities of its members working in the Medical School, the Health Professions Council and the Ministry of Health and Child Welfare. Doctors continue to exercise dominance over other workers, partly because the regulatory system, which is a carry-over from the colonial period, has not been restructured since independence. Inadequate monitoring of doctors has left them with more clinical and economic autonomy than they should have. In addition, the medical profession has been able to maintain its dominance due to the role played by doctors in the Ministry of Health and in the Health Professions Council, thus confirming Bjorkman's (1989) point regarding the role of bureaucratic professionals in maintaining autonomy. Thus, the nature of medical autonomy and dominance in Zimbabwe and the factors which account for its erosion or maintenance are different from those existing in Britain and the United States.

The findings of this study confirm Freidson's (1989) third point, that salaried employment is not incompatible with professional dominance and that the latter is determined more by the value of the goods and services offered to the society rather than by the profession's employment status. The services of government-employed doctors at the Parirenyatwa Group of Hospitals are highly valued and they themselves enjoy high social esteem, as evidenced by, among other things, the influence which they are able to exert in negotiating their conditions of employment. We noted that in the Zimbabwean case, the strongest threat to medical autonomy arises from shortage of resources and breakdowns of equipment.

In response to Freidson's fourth point we noted earlier in this chapter, that the advisory style of management prevails at the Parirenyatwa Group of Hospitals and, to date no attempt has been made to introduce strict medical practice guidelines comparable to those introduced in the United States. While the government is still concerned with ensuring that all its citizens have access to health care, the quality of that care has not been seriously addressed.

Freidson's medical dominance theory is pertinent for analysing the nature of medical autonomy in Zimbabwe because it is the most comprehensive to date. In addition, as one of the aims of this study is to offer some comparisons of the nature of medical autonomy in Zimbabwe with that in other contexts, it is necessary to rely on global concepts in the analysis of medical autonomy. But as we have seen from the above arguments, the theory cannot adequately explain the nature of medical autonomy in Zimbabwe because it is based on developments in the United States, which differ significantly from those under analysis in this thesis. Just as there are differences in the emergence of the medical profession in Zimbabwe and in the description given by Freidson, so do the factors that account for the maintenance and erosion of autonomy differ in the different contexts. We noted that although the medical profession continues to enjoy medical autonomy in the post-colonial era, the professional associations, which are weak and ineffective, have done little to protect or extend it. Medical autonomy in the post-colonial era has been maintained as a result of the threat by junior doctors to withdraw their labour, the opposition of the private economic sector and international finance institutions to policies which are inimical to medicine's and their interests. As mentioned earlier in this chapter, the medical profession has been able to exercise a relatively high degree of autonomy by default, i.e. as a result of poor monitoring and regulation of the profession by the responsible institutions and personnel. Although Freidson's dominance theory is the most comprehensive to date, it is of limited viability in analysing professions in other societies because of its Anglo-American focus. Attempts to reduce its parochiality have seen its application in continental Europe (Garpenby, 1989; Riska, 1988), but to date, there has been no significant attempt to extend it to developing countries, and the same limitation applies to the deprofessionalisation hypothesis discussed below.

Deprofessionalisation Hypothesis

Maria Haug (1973, 1988) claims that the medical profession is losing its societal position marked with prestige and trust. Firstly, she argues that its monopoly over medical knowledge is being undermined by the increasing use of automated retrieval systems, such as computerised algorithms for symptom assessment. Secondly, the increasingly educated and critical general public is less likely to regard medical knowledge as esoteric and is much more inclined to challenge the doctor's authority in the treatment process. Thirdly, the fact that much medical work now takes place in teams, including non-physician experts, on whom physicians have to rely, reduces medical dominance. Fourthly, the increase of consumer self-help groups is seen as spearheading the consumer revolt and increasing reliance on alternative health workers. Fifthly, and finally, Haug argues that escalating health costs have damaged doctors' altruistic public image.

The nature of medical autonomy prevailing at the Parirenyatwa Group of Hospitals does not confirm the assertions of the deprofessionalisation hypothesis. With respect to the first point raised by Haug, computers are a very scarce commodity in Zimbabwe, both for members of the general public and government hospitals. To date, there have certainly been no attempts to use computers for purposes stated by the deprofessionalisation hypothesis. With regards to the second point above, we noted that there is a big information gap between practitioners and the majority of their clients about health care in general and the treatment process, including its likely outcome, in particular. Most patients treated at the Parirenyatwa Group of Hospitals are not assertive and are highly unlikely to challenge the doctors' authority in treatment. They tend to leave the decision-making concerning their treatment to their doctors which gives the latter more discretion in their work than their counterparts in developed countries. With respect to the third point concerning medical teamwork, doctors in Zimbabwe retain their dominance even when they work as members of a team comprising some non-medical experts. With regards to the fourth point, our findings indicate that in Zimbabwe there are no significant self-help groups, feminist or consumer organisations specifically aimed at improving the quality of health care or holding health care providers accountable for their work.

We further noted that although traditional healers are widely consulted, they do not pose a challenge to medical dominance because they are consulted for specific medical conditions and are not recognised for health insurance purposes or for official certification. In any case, they operate outside the structures of the formal health service. With reference to the final point raised by Haug, although health costs have gone up, they are largely blamed on the Government and international finance institutions rather than doctors. From this evidence, we can conclude that the assumptions of the deprofessionalisation hypothesis have no validity to the analysis of medical autonomy in the Zimbabwean context. The deprofessionalisation hypothesis, like the proletarianisation hypothesis discussed below, was aimed at supplanting dominance theory, it also has been limited to examination of the Anglo-American phenomenon.

Proletarianisation Hypothesis

McKinlay and Arches (1985, 1986) and McKinlay and Stoeckle (1986) hold that the growing corporatization and bureaucratization of medicine is significantly curtailing the autonomy which physicians used to exercise in a number of areas of their work, including the location and content of that work, remuneration of labour and medical education. Secondly, they argue that doctors are increasingly being subjected to more exacting control in their work place, and that even though the managers in health organisations are often doctors, they act in the interests of the organisation rather than of the profession. These theorists contend that under these conditions the medical profession cannot be described as professionally dominant.

Contrary to the assertions of the proletarianisation hypothesis, the evidence presented in this thesis suggests that government-employed doctors at the Parirenyatwa Group of Hospitals enjoy more economic autonomy than one would expect of salaried employees. With regard to the first point, doctors cannot determine the location of the government hospitals in which they work, but we have noted that they have successfully challenged Government's right to place them at less desirable rural institutions. They also defeated Government's attempt, through the abortive Health Institutions and Services Bill (1989), to determine where they can locate their private medical offices. In terms of ability to determine their remuneration, we noted that government-employed doctors have more leverage in negotiating their conditions of service and have done much better in this respect than any other health workers. Consultants have been given the right to treat their private patients in and outside government hospitals and no serious regulatory mechanisms have been put in place to ensure that they work according to the terms of their contracts.

It is conceivable that as the opportunities for working in neighbouring countries decrease and the private medical sector in Zimbabwe gets saturated, government-employed doctors may find it more difficult to determine their remuneration to the same extent as at present, particularly taking into account the recently doubled medical school intake. With regard to the second point raised by the proletarianisation argument, doctors in Zimbabwe are still subject to an advisory type of management rather than the authoritative and prescriptive type which has been held responsible for eroding medical autonomy in the United States. Evidence from this thesis suggests that medical professionals in administrative positions continue to identify with the rank and file, partly because of the high turnover in the administrative positions but also because doctors in Zimbabwe are a very small community. This makes professional stratification on that basis highly unlikely in the foreseeable future. In conclusion, we can say that most of the assertions of the advocates of the proletarianisation hypothesis are not confirmed by the findings of this study, although it is possible that some of them may emerge in the future. Although the proletarianisation hypothesis is ethnocentric in its focus, it is of some relevance because it examines the nature of medical autonomy for salaried professionals employed in bureaucratic organisations, which has been the focus of this study. However, Johnson's model of the medical profession in post-colonial states discussed below is much more relevant for analysing the Zimbabwean context.

Johnson's Model of Professions in Colonial and Post-colonial States

Firstly, Johnson (1972, 1973) argues that the historical, cultural, social and political circumstances prevailing in Third world countries were and remain inimical to the development of professionalism, which was a historically and culturally bound occurrence. Consequently, professions in Third world countries emerged from and remain embedded in social structures and power relations which are essentially different from those in Britain and the United States, and gave rise to corporate patronage rather than professionalism. With corporate patronage, a powerful client regulates the provider rather than the profession itself. The most important demand for professional services was from the colonial administration, which defined its needs and the way they were to be met.

Secondly, Johnson (1973) maintains that even though some of the outward manifestations of professionalism are present, these lack its essential attributes. For example, even though there are professional associations, these are weak and have not developed their own code of behaviour and, as a result professionals have not internalised the essential attributes of professionalism. The associations do not control medical education, which is the responsibility of a government or another agency responsible to it, instead, they are more concerned with fighting for conditions of service for members. Thirdly, Johnson (1973) considered it highly unlikely that there could be a heterogenous group of middle class people demanding private medical services in a post-colonial state. In any case, setting up a private practice depends on the patronage of administrative officials.

With regard to the first point, Johnson is obviously correct that the historical, cultural, social and political circumstances prevailing in post-colonial states are different from those which existed in Britain and the United States of America when medicine emerged as a profession. Similarly, Johnson's point that the social structures and power relations prevailing in these states continue to be different from those of developed countries is valid as we noted in Chapter 1. However, Rhodesia was not just a colony, but a white settler state which attempted to recreate the same environment that existed in Britain. We found that the medical profession was not only there to meet the needs of the administrative personnel, as was the case in other colonies, but that there was a large population of independent settlers demanding private medical services. Most of the doctors were, in fact, settlers themselves and expected to live and work in Rhodesia for the rest of their lives. With regards to the second point raised by Johnson, we saw in Chapter 3 that the medical profession in Rhodesia had a different relationship with the colonial administration from that described by Johnson (1973). Contrary to Johnson's assertion, doctors enjoyed a high degree of autonomy in all aspects of their work and the professional association actively fought to protect and extend it. However, after independence, there were countervailing factors which prevented the state from passing policies which could erode medical autonomy, which include the Lancaster House Constitution, a large white population, a dynamic private economic sector, international finance institutions and donor countries, all of which ensured that the post-colonial government could not change the prevailing situation too radically and undermine existing institutions. For example, government's expressed intention to abolish private medicine met with serious opposition from these countervailing forces and the abandonment of this policy enabled the medical profession to retain its economic autonomy.

Johnson is correct in pointing out that the professional associations in post-colonial states are weak and lack the legal and organisational capacity to play the role which they did during the period of professionalisation in developed countries and continue to play in those countries today. In spite of the weakness of its associations, the medical profession in Zimbabwe continues to exercise autonomy in the various aspects of its work, mainly due to the ineffectiveness of the existing regulatory structures and due to the efforts of its members working in the Ministry of Health and the Health Professions Council. The ineffectiveness of the regulatory structures is itself a function of the disjuncture between, on one hand, the post-colonial state and, its administrative apparatus based on rational-legal principles and, on the other, the wider society over which it presides.

Johnson's (1973) third point, concerning lack of opportunities for private practice, is not confirmed by events in Zimbabwe where there has always existed a viable private medical sector, which enables doctors to practise privately either on a part-time or full-time basis without relying on administrative patronage. One of the reasons given for the rejection of the Health Services and Institutions Bill (1989) by the medical profession was the latter's fear that the Minister of Health could use the powers conferred on him or her by the bill in a nepotistic manner. As we saw, the medical profession was able to defeat the bill because of countervailing forces which forced government to retain the *status quo*. There is evidence of nepotism in Zimbabwe, as we noted earlier, but it is difficult to estimate how prevalent the practise is.

Johnson's conceptualisation of professions in post-colonial states is relevant to the analysis of the Zimbabwean situation simply because it is alone in recognising the uniqueness of professions in Third World countries and post-colonial states in particular. However, his characterisation is somewhat out of date and has become increasingly less viable as an analytical tool because it was conceived almost a quarter of a century ago, just under a decade before Zimbabwe became independent. At the time most of the post-colonial states were in their first decade of independence and the socio-economic and political landscape has since changed significantly for most. His analysis took place during the era of the one-party state in Africa, and although then newly independent, most were in effect in rather better

232

economic shape at that time than they are today. The 1980s and 1990s have seen serious economic deterioration, with most African countries becoming more reliant on conditional foreign aid than ever before, as well as political upheavals which have seen the demise of the one party state system and in some, the emergence of fragile democracies. A new characterisation of medical autonomy which takes this new scenario into account is thus long over due.

Towards a Model of Medical Autonomy in Post-colonial States in Africa

From the findings of the book it is possible to propose a model of medical autonomy in post-colonial states which is both descriptive and explanatory. The model describes the significant features of medical practice at present and, more importantly, also explains the existence of those features, identifying the key underlying factors and processes. The medical profession in post-colonial states in Africa emerged under unique historical, political, economic, social and cultural circumstances, as pointed out by Johnson (1973). Specifically, the factors which continue to shape medical autonomy differ significantly from those discussed by current theories of professions for western developed countries. The factors influencing medical autonomy in Africa are: the persistence of pre-industrial cultural values in the wider society; severe national economic crises; and the influence of international donor countries and finance organisations.

Persistence of Pre-industrial Cultural Values

The medical profession was parachuted into Africa, along with other institutions intended to meet the needs of the colonial administration and settlers. Even though an attempt was made to recreate the professional conditions existing in the colonizing countries, the medical profession evolved quite differently. During the colonial era, most doctors worked as salaried employees in state-run health institutions and there were very few opportunities for carrying out private medical practice in most countries because most of the patients were poor. The regulation of medical education, licensing and discipline was the responsibility of a government department or institution dominated by the medical profession.

The colonial administrative structures, including those responsible for medical regulation were based on rational-legal principles which also underpin the cultural values of the Anglo-American societies. During the colonial era, the administrators, the medical profession and the immigrant population shared the same cultural values. There was, therefore, minimum malfunctioning of the administrative structures attributable to cultural differences, although these did arise when dealing with the indigenous population. The indigenization of administrative structures which occurred after independence in most African countries meant that the cultural beliefs of administrators, the professionals and the wider society were largely those of pre-industrial societies, while the administrative structures, including those responsible for regulating the medical profession remained the same, i.e. based on rational-legal authority. One of the main reasons for the lack of assimilation of rational-legal principles was the lack of preparation of the indigenous administration by colonialists before the handover at independence. In Western developed countries, bureaucratic administrative structures evolved over a long period with the society and are ingrained in their cultural and social values. In pre-industrial societies, on the other hand, authority rests in the person and not the office which they hold, as suggested by Weber (1978), and public office is used in pursuit of private goals, giving rise to patrimonialism. Loyalty to one's kin is of more primary value than efficiency for the public good. Not surprisingly, the inherited administrative and regulatory structures were hit by functional problems, including paralysing patrimonial practices, because public transparency and accountability were not ingrained in the pre-industrial value system. Those in senior political or administrative positions often facilitate contravention of laid down administrative procedures by their junior employees who are their kin, thereby not only setting a bad precedent, but also undermining the authority of the person in charge. Poor assimilation and identification with the principles underlying most of the administrative structures results in inadequate professional regulation, which in turn enables, by default, government-employed doctors to exercise higher autonomy than they should.

National Economic Crises

After independence most of the African states embarked on large-scale expansion of social services such as health care to meet the needs of the previously neglected indigenous population. This expansion which marked the first decade of independence of most African countries was, however, not matched by economic growth. Much of the expansion was funded from government revenue and foreign donations and loans but by the mid-1980s most African countries were experiencing incapacitating fiscal deficits as a result of world recession, heavy external debts, shrinking donor funds, misuse of funds but, in some cases, due to wanton looting of public funds by the political leaders. Some of the most telling evidence of the declining economies lies in the deterioration of social services, including health care, evident in the breakdown of physical infrastructure and equipment, shortage of almost all types resources and shortages of doctors in government hospitals.

Most African governments had no option but to adopt IMF/World Bank initiated economic structural adjustment programmes aimed at rescuing their ailing economies. This entails: cutting back on expenditure on social services like health and education; cost sharing for government and users; removal of economic and social subsidies; and opening up most sectors to private enterprise, thus opening up the market for private medical services.

In most African countries, the state is the biggest provider of health services and the biggest employer of health professionals including doctors. Thus, the declining national economic performance hits doctors in both their professional and personal capacity. Reduction of the health budget aggravates the crippling shortages of resources, such as equipment and even basic drugs like analgesics, hitting the poor who cannot afford private health facilities hardest. Shortage and the unavailability of necessary health resources seriously constrains doctors' clinical performance and affects the outcome of medical intervention leading to frustration and demoralisation. The doctors' frustration is compounded by the fact that a large number of patients attending government hospitals could have been successfully treated if the resources were available, or if they were able to pay for them.

The deteriorating economic situation leads to downward spiralling of incomes, a declining standard of living and escalating costs, making economic survival an uphill struggle for most people, including doctors. When the government health institutions were well equipped and resourced, the majority of the population preferred them because they charged sub-economic rates, and consequently private medical practice was not a viable option for most doctors. The latter, like other workers react by engaging in extra economic survival strategies outside their regular employment. With the deterioration of government hospitals, the public, including former non-paying patients are reduced to hospital shopping in search of those with resources, even if it means paying much more for treatment. This has not only stopped those better able to pay for medical care from going to public hospitals, thus further starving the hospitals of badly needed funds, but it has also created a market for private medical practice. In order to take advantage of this opportunity of supplementing their government income, doctors manipulate their government work schedule and work in their private offices during normal working hours after rushing through the normal work schedule, doing the bare minimum or not turning up for work at all. Those without private offices may take on locum duties during working hours, evenings or weekends, depending on the available options. Some migrate to other countries where conditions of service are better. Others may go into business ventures which are not in any way related to medicine, such as supermarkets, automobile service stations, for example.

The struggle for economic survival has contributed to the ineffectiveness of the medical regulatory structures. Those charged with regulating doctors have seen their own wages declining and usually engage in their own economic survival strategies, understand the behaviour of the doctors and do not sanction them. As this process involves all grades of doctors, all of them end up with more clinical and economic autonomy than they should have, by default.

The Countervailing Impact of Foreign Governments and Donor Agencies

Another feature which is unique to developing and post-colonial states is the presence of external forces in the form of international finance institutions and donor countries. Most former colonies have, since independence, relied on loans and grants either from foreign governments or finance institutions such as the World Bank and the International Monetary Fund (IMF). Some of the loans and grants were used in the provision of social services and other public projects, but most of this did not create national wealth. Before the world recession and the collapse of the former Eastern block, African countries could secure substantial funds fairly easily and, by the mid-1980s most found themselves encumbered with heavy external debts, some of them unsustainable. Even under the best of circumstances, external aid comes with certain conditionalities which constrain both internal and external policies of the recipient country. For example, donor countries and institutions can dictate that the donor funds are only used in promotion of the private sector or that they will only release the funds if democratic elections are held or after certain corrupt officials have been removed from government office. By the same token, they can threaten to withdraw or withhold aid if the conditionalities are not met or if the government is disagreeable in any way. Foreign aid agencies are succeeding in making authoritarian and formerly unresponsive governments responsive and permeable to their citizens to an extent.

With the collapse of the former Eastern block and the current demand for acceptable human rights records, pluralist government, transparency and accountability, most post-colonial countries find that foreign aid has shrunk drastically and the conditionalities are more intrusive to both internal and external policies. Civil groups in post-colonial countries often appeal to donor countries and agencies to withhold aid from their governments in order to force them to abandon or fulfil certain conditions. The demise of the once popular one-party state in Africa has been attributed to aid granting conditionalities. Most of the economic structural adjustment programmes, which have wrecked havoc on most post-colonial economies and brought such untold suffering, in some cases resulting in the fall of governments, are another testimony to the salience of foreign donor agencies on the sovereignty of these countries and their internal social dynamics. The countervailing effect of donor agencies on state autonomy seriously affects the relationship of the state and civil groups in the country. For example, encouraging cost-sharing in the health sector and the development of the private health sector enhances doctors' economic autonomy. The reality is that post-colonial and other developing countries have to contend with strong external countervailing forces which have a significant impact on medical autonomy, a situation which does not arise in western developed countries.

Directions for Future Research

This book has shown that doctors in Zimbabwe, a post-colonial state, enjoy considerable autonomy in their work and at the same time, has highlighted the fact that the factors which maintain or erode medical autonomy in this society are different from those discussed by the current theories of professions. The above review of current competing theories of professions clearly exposes their ethnocentric nature, being firmly based on the characterisation of the medical profession in the Anglo-American context, with none capturing the distinctive nature of medical autonomy in post-colonial states. It is hoped that the model of medical autonomy in post-colonial states in Africa presented above will form the basis of future research and that the characterisation, which represents an extension of current theories of professions, will be taken into account in the conception of more inclusive theories of professions.

Bibliography

Books and Articles

Agere, S.T. (1986), 'Progress and Problems in the Health Care Delivery System', in I. Mandaza (ed), *The Political Economy of Transition 1980-1986*, pp. 355-378, CODESRIA, Dakar.

Alaszewski, A. (1995), 'Restructuring Health and Welfare Professions in the United Kingdom: The Impact of Internal Markets on the Medical, Nursing and Social Work Professions', in T. Johnson, G. Larkin and M. Saks (eds), *Health Professions and the State in Europe*, pp. 55-74, Routledge, London.

Alford, R.A. (1975), *Health Care Politics*, University of Chicago Press, Chicago.

Allen, I. (1994), *Doctors and their Careers: A New Generation*, Policy Studies Institute, London.

Annandale, E. (1989), 'Proletarianisation or Restratification of the Medical Profession? The Case of Obstetrics', *International Journal of Health Services*, 19 (4), pp. 611-634.

Atkinson, P. (1981), *The Clinical Experience: The Construction and Reconstruction of Medical Reality*, Gower, Aldershot.

Barnes, J.A. (1979), *Who Should Know What?*, Penguin, Harmondsworth.

Bell, J. (1993), *Doing Your Research Project*, Open University Press, Buckingham.

Bjorkman, J.W. (1989), 'Politicizing Medicine and Medicalising Politics: Physician Power in the United States', in G. Freddi and J.W. Bjorkman (eds), *Controlling Medical Professionals*, pp. 28-73, Sage Publications, London.

Bloom, G. (1985), 'Two Models for Change in the Health Services in Zimbabwe', *International Journal of Health Services*, 15 (3), pp. 451-468.

Blumer, M. (1984), *Sociological Research Methods: An Introduction*, Second Edition, The Macmillan Press Ltd, London.

Bottomore, T. (1993), *Elites and Society*, Second Edition, Routledge, London.

Bourdillon, M.F.C. (1987), *The Shona Peoples*, Third Edition, Mambo Press, Gweru.

Burgess, R. (1982), 'Multiple Strategies in Field Research', in R. G. Burgess (ed), *Field Research: A Sourcebook and Field Manual*, pp. 163-167, Routledge, London.

British Medical Association (1958), 'The Approaching Retirement of Dr. R.M. Morris', *Central African Journal of Medicine*, April, pp. 171-174.

Bryman, A. (1988), *Quantity and Quality in Social Research*, Unwin Hyman, London.

Callaghy, T.M. (1988), 'The State and the Development of Capitalism in Africa: Theoretical, Historical and Comparative Reflections', in D. Rothchild and N. Chazan (eds), *The Precarious Balance: State and Society in Africa*, pp. 67-99, Westview Press, Boulder.

Chakaodza, A.M. (1993), *Structural Adjustment in Zambia and Zimbabwe*, Third World Publishing House, Harare.

Chanfreau, D. (1979), 'Professional Ideology and the Health Care System in Chile', *International Journal of Health Services*, 9 (1).

Chavunduka, G. L. (1988), 'The Organisation of Traditional Medicine in Zimbabwe', in M. Last and G. Chavunduka (eds), *Professionalisation of African Medicine*, pp. 29-50, Manchester University Press in Association with International African Institute, Manchester.

Chavunduka, G.L. (1978), *Traditional Healers and the Shona Patient*, Mambo Press, Gweru.

Chazan, N., Mortimer, R., Ravenhill, J. and Rothchild, D. (1992), *Politics and Society in Contemporary Africa*, Second Edition, Lynne Rienner Publishers, Boulder.

Chibwe, C. & Bwalya, J. M. (1990), 'Zambia', in V. Subramaniam (ed), *Public Administration in the Third World*, pp. 289-308, Greenwood Press, West Port.

Clapham, C. (1985), *Third World Politics*, London, Routledge.

Clarke, D.G. (1977), *Agricultural and Plantation Workers in Rhodesia*, Mambo Press, Gweru.

Coburn, D. (1988), 'Canadian Medicine: Dominance or Proletarianisation', *The Milbank Quarterly*, 66 (Supplement 2), pp. 92-116.

Coburn, D. (1992), 'Freidson Then and Now: An 'Internalist' Critique of Freidson's Past and Present Views of the Medical Profession', *International Journal of Health Services*, 22 (3), pp. 497-512.

Cohen, E. (1979), The Report of the Committee formed to Investigate the Future of Medicine Under African Majority Rule, (unpublished), Harare.

Cowen, M.B. (1995), *A Central African Odyssey*, The Radcliffe Press, London.

Davies, R. (1988), 'The Transition To Socialism in Zimbabwe, Some Areas of Debate', in C. Stoneman (ed), *Zimbabwe's Prospects*, pp. 18-42, Macmillan, London.

Dent, M. (1995), 'Doctors, Peer Review and Quality Assurance', in T. Johnson, G. Larkin and M. Saks (eds), *Health Professions and the State in Europe*, pp. 86-102, Routledge, London.

Denzin, N.K. (1989), *The Research Act*, Third Edition, Prentice Hall International, London.

Derber, C., Schwartz, W.A. and Magrass, Y. (1990), *Power in the Highest Degree, Professionals and the Rise of the New Mandarin Order*, Oxford University Press, Oxford.

Derbyshire J.D. and Patterson D.T. (1979), *An Introduction to Public Administration*, McGraw-Hill, London.

Dey, I. (1993), *Qualitative Data Analysis*, London, Routledge.

Doyal, L and Pennell, I. (1979), *The Political Economy of Health*, Pluto Press, London.

Doyal, L. (1994), 'Changing Medicine? Gender and the Politics of Health Care', in J.Gabe, D. Kelleher and G. Williams (eds), *Challenging Medicine*, pp. 140-159, Routledge, London.

Dohler, M. (1989), 'Physicians' Professional Autonomy in the Welfare States: Endangered or Preserved?', in G. Freddi and J.W. Bjorkman (eds), *Controlling Medical Professions*, pp. 178-197, Sage Publications, London.

Elston, M. (1977), 'Medical Autonomy: Challenge and Response', in K. Barnard and K. Lee (eds), *Conflicts in the National Health Service*, pp. 26-51, Croom Helm, London.

Elston, M. A. (1991), 'The Politics of Professional Power: Medicine in the Changing Health Service', in J. Gabe, M. Calnan and M. Bury (eds), *The Sociology of the Health Service*, pp. 58-87, Routledge, London.

Esterday, L. (1982), 'The Making of a Female Researcher: Role Problems in Fieldwork', in R.G. Burgess (ed), *Field Research: A Soucebook and Field Manual*, pp. 62-67, Routledge, London.

Feltoe, G. and Nyapadi, T.J. (1989), *Law and Medicine in Zimbabwe*, Baobab Books in Association with the Legal Resources Foundation, Harare.

Fenn, P. and Dingwall, R. (1992), 'The Tort System and Information: Some Comparisons Between U.K. and U.S.', in R. Dingwall and P. Fenn (eds), *Quality and Regulation in Health Care*, pp. 11-25, Routledge, London.

Fielding, N. (1982), 'Observational Research on the National Front', in M. Bulmer (ed), *Social Research Ethics*, Macmillan, London.

Fielding, N. (1993), 'Qualitative Interviewing', in N. Gilbert (ed), *Researching Social Life*, pp. 135-153, Sage Publications Ltd, London.

Fielding, N. (1993), 'Ethnography', in N. Gilbert (ed), *Researching Social Life*, pp. 154-171, Sage Publications, London.

Forsyth G. (1973), *Doctors and State Medicine*, London, Pitman.

Fraser Ross, W. (1975), 'Medical Training in Rhodesia', *Central African Journal of Medicine*, 21 (11), pp. 34-40.

Fraser Ross, W. 'Rhodesian Doctors', *Central African Journal of Medicine*, 13 (12), pp. 273-280.

Freddi, G. (1989), 'Problems of Organisational Rationality in Health Systems: Political Controls and Policy Options', in G. Freddi and J.W. Bjorkman (eds), *Controlling Medical Professionals*, pp. 1-27, Sage Publications, London.

Friedson E. (1988), *Profession of Medicine*, Second Edition, The University of Chicago Press, Chicago.

Friedson, E. (1989a), 'The Reorganisation of the Medical Profession', in *Medical Work in America*, pp. 178-205, Yale University Press, New Haven.

Freidson, E. (1989b), *Medical Work in America*, Yale University Press, New Haven.

Freidson, E. (1994), *Professionalism Reborn*, Polity Press, Cambridge.

Frenk, J. and Durans-Arenas, L. (1993), 'The Medical Profession and the State', in F.W. Hafferty and J.B. McKinlay (eds), *The Changing Medical Profession*, pp. 25-42, Oxford University Press, Oxford.

Gann, L.H. and Gelfand, M. (1964), *Huggins of Rhodesia*, George Allen and Unwin Ltd., London.

Gans, H.J. (1982), 'The Participant Observer as a Human Being: Observations on the Personal Aspects of Fieldwork', in R.G. Burgess (ed), *Field Research: A Sourcebook and Field Manual*, pp. 53-61, Routledge, London.

Garfield R. and Williams G. (1989), *The Nicaraguan Experience*, Oxfam, Oxford.

Garpenby, P. (1989), *The State and the Medical Profession: A Cross-national Comparison of the Health Policy Arena in the UK and Sweden*, University of Linkoping, Linkoping.

Gelfand, M. (1972), 'Whither Medicine in the Next Five Years', *Central African Journal of Medicine*, 18 (4), pp. 80-85.

Gelfand, M. (1975), 'The Future Doctors of Rhodesia', *Central African Journal of Medicine*, 21 (11), pp. 238-243.

Gelfand, M. (1953), *Tropical Victory*, Cape Town, Juta & Co.

Gelfand, M. (1976), *A Service to the Sick*, Mambo Press, Gwelo.

Gelfand, M. (ed), (1959), *The Fleming Letters (1894-1914)*, The Central African Journal of Medicine, Medical Books Department, Salisbury.

Gelfand, M. (1988), *Godly Medicine in Zimbabwe*, Mambo Press, Gweru.

Gilmurray, J., Riddell, R. and Sanders, D. (1979), *The Struggle for Health*, Mambo Press, Gwelo.

Gish, O. (1971), *Doctor Migration and World Health*, G. Bell and Sons, London.

Gish, O. and Martin, G. (1979), 'A Reappraisal of the 'Brain Drain' with Special Reference to the Medical Profession', *Social Science and Medicine*, 13 (c), pp. 1-11.

Glaser, B.G. and Strauss, A.L. (1967), *The Discovery of Grounded Theory: Strategies for Qualitative Research*, Aldine, Chicago.

Globerman, J. (1990), 'Free Enterprise, Professional Ideology, and Self-Interest: An Evaluation of Resistance by Canadian Physicians to Universal Health Insurance', *Journal of Health and Social Behaviour*, 31, pp. 11-27.

Gyimah-Boadi, E. and Rothchild, D. (1990), 'Ghana', in V. Subramaniam (ed), *Public Administration in the Third World*, pp. 229-277, Greenwood Press, West Port.

Hafferty, F.W. and Light, D.W. (1995), 'Professional Dynamics and the Changing Nature of Medical Work', *Journal of Health and Social Behaviour*, Extra Issue, pp. 132-153.

Hafferty, F.W. and McKinlay, J.B. (eds), *The Changing Medical Profession*, Oxford University Press, Oxford.

242

Hafferty, F.W. and Wolinsky, F.D. (1991), 'Conflicting Characterisations of Professional Dominance', *Current Research on Occupations and Professions*, 6, pp. 225-249.

Hammersley, M. and Atkinson, P. (1983), *Ethnography: Principles in Practice*, Routledge, London.

Hanlon, J. (1988), 'Destabilisation and the Battle to Reduce Dependence', in C. Stoneman (ed), *Zimbabwe's Prospects*, pp. 32-42, Macmillan Publishers, London.

Harrison, S. and Schulz, R.I. (1989), 'Clinical Autonomy in the United Kingdom and the United States: Contrasts and Convergence', in G. Freddi and J.W. Bjorkman (eds), *Controlling Medical Professionals*, Sage Publications, London.

Haug, M.R.A. (1973), 'Deprofessionalisation: An Alternate Hypothesis for the Future', *The Sociological Review Monograph*, 20, pp. 195-211.

Haug, M.R.A. (1988), 'Re-examination of the Hypothesis of Physician Deprofessionalisation', *The Milbank Quarterly*, 66 (Supplement 2), pp. 48-56.

Hawkins, A. M. (1993), 'The State and the Post-independence Economy of Zimbabwe', Unpublished paper.

Herbst, J. (1990), *The State and Policy Making in Zimbabwe*, University of Zimbabwe Press, Harare.

Hill, M.R. (1993), *Archival Strategies and Techniques*, Sage Publications, London.

Hodder-Williams, R. (1984), *An Introduction to the Politics of Tropical Africa*, George Allen & Unwin, London.

Honigmann, J.J. (1982), 'Sampling in Ethnographic Fieldwork', in R.G. Burgess (ed), *Field Research: A Sourcebook and Manual*, pp. 79-90, Routledge, London.

Hornsby-Smith, M. (1993), 'Gaining Access', in Gilbert, N. (ed), *Researching Social Life*, Sage Publications, London.

Hugman, R. (1991), *Power in Caring Professions*, Macmillan, Houndsmill.

Hunter, D.J. (1994), 'From Tribalism to Corporatism', in J. Gabe, D. Kelleher and G. Williams (eds), *Challenging Medicine*, pp. 1-22, Routledge, London.

Illich, I. (1976), *Limits to Medicine*, Penguin, Harmondsworth.

Johnson, T.J. and Caygill, M. (1972), 'Community in the Making: Aspects of Britain's Role in the Development of Professional Education in the Commonwealth', Unpublished.

243

Johnson, T. (1972), *Professions and Power*, Macmillan, London.

Johnson T. (1973), 'Imperialism and the Professions', *The Sociological Review Monograph*, 20, pp. 281-309.

Johnson, T. (1995), 'Governmentality and the Institutionalisation of Expertise', in T. Johnson, G. Larkin and M. Saks (eds), *Health Professions and the State in Europe*, pp. 7-22, Routledge, London.

Kelleher, D. (1994), 'Self-help Groups and their Relationship to Medicine', in J. Gabe, D. Kelleher and G. Williams (eds), *Challenging Medicine*, pp. 104-117, Routledge, London.

Kelleher, D., Gabe, J. and Williams, G. (1994), 'Understanding Medical Dominance in the Modern World', in J. Gabe, D. Keller and G. Williams (eds), *Challenging Medicine*, pp. xii-xxix, Routledge, London.

Klein, R. (1989), *The Politics of the National Health Service*, Second Edition, Longman Group, London.

Larkin, G.V. (1983), *Occupational Monopoly and Modern Medicine*, Tavistock, London.

Larkin, S.V. (1988), 'Medical Dominance in Britain: Image and Historical Reality', *The Milbank Quarterly*, 66 (Supplement 2), pp. 117-152.

Larkin, G. (1995), 'State Control and the Health Professions in the United Kingdom, Historical Perspectives', in T. Johnson, G. Larkin and M. Saks (eds), *Health Professions and the State in Europe*, pp. 45-54, Routledge, London.

Lee, R.M. (1993), *Doing Research on Sensitive Topics*, Sage Publications, London.

Lee, R.M. and Renzetti, C. M. (1993), 'The Problems of Researching Sensitive Topics', in C.M. Renzetti and R.M. Lee (eds), *Researching Sensitive Topics*, Sage Publications, London.

Lennock, J. (1994), *Poverty and Structural Adjustment in Zimbabwe*, Oxfam Publications, Oxford.

Levy, L.F. (1961), 'The Way to Remedy the Present Shortage of Doctors', *Central African Journal of Medicine*, January, pp. 31-32.

Light, D.W. (1988), 'Turf Battles and the Theory of Professional Dominance', *Research in the Sociology of Health Care*, 7, pp. 203-225.

Light, D.W. (1991), 'Conflicting Characterisations of Professional Dominance', *Current Research on Occupations and Professions*, 6, pp. 225-249.

Light, D. (1995), 'Countervailing Powers: A Framework for Professions in Transition', in T. Johnson, G. Larkin and M. Saks (eds), *Health Professions and the State in Europe*, pp. 25-41, Routledge, London.

Light, D.W. (1993), 'Countervailing Power: The Changing Character of the Medical Profession in the United States', in F.W. Hafferty and J.B. McKinlay (eds), *The Changing Medical Profession: An International Perspective*, pp. 69-79, Oxford University Press, New York.

Light, D. and Levine, S. (1988), 'The Changing Character of the Medical Profession: A Theoretical Overview', *The Milbank Quarterly*, 66 (Supplement 2), pp. 10-32.

Loewenson, R. (1991), 'Health and Health Care in Post-independence Rural Zimbabwe', in N.D. Mutizwa-Mangiza and A.H.J. Helmsing (eds), *Rural Development and Planning in Zimbabwe*, pp. 360-381, Avebury, Aldershot.

Loewenson, R. and Sanders, D. (1988), 'The Political Economy of Health and Nutrition', in C. Stoneman (ed), *Zimbabwe's Prospects*, pp. 133-152, Macmillan, London.

Loewenson, R. (1990), 'An Overview of Health Manpower Issues in Relation to Equity in Health Services in Zimbabwe', *Journal of Social Development in Africa*, 5 (1), pp. 23-29.

Lofland, J. and Lofland L.H. (1984), *Analysing Social Settings*, Second Edition, Wandsworth Publishing Company, Belmont.

Mandaza, I. (1987), 'The State and Politics in the Post-White Settler Colonial Situation', in I. Mandaza (ed), *Zimbabwe: The Political Economy of Transition, 1980-1986*, pp. 21-74, CODESRIA, Kent.

Mandaza, I. (1991), 'The One Party State and Democracy in Southern Africa: Towards a Conceptual Framework', in I. Mandaza and L.M. Sachikonye (eds), *The One Party State and Democracy: The Zimbabwe Debate*, pp. 19-41, Southern Africa Political Economy (SAPES) Trust, Harare.

Manga, P. (1988), 'The Transformation of Zimbabwe's Health Care: A Review of the White Paper on Health', *Social Science and Medicine*, 27 (11), pp. 1131-1138.

McKinlay, J.B. (1973), 'On the Professional Regulation of Change', *Sociological Review Monograph*, 20, pp. 61-81.

McKinlay, J.B. (1988), 'The Changing Character of the Medical Profession', *The Milbank Quarterly*, 66 (Supplement 2), pp. 1-9.

McKinlay, J.B. and Arches J. (1986), 'Historical Changes in Doctoring: A Reply to Milton Roemer', *International Journal of Health Services*, 16 (3), pp. 473-477.

McKinlay, J.B. and Arches, J. (1985), 'Towards the Proletarianisation of Physicians', *International Journal of Health Services*, 15 (2), pp. 161-195.

McKinlay, J.B. and Stoeckle, J.D. (1988), 'Corporatisation and the Social Transformation of Doctoring', *International Journal of Health Services*, 18 (2), pp. 191-205.

Miles, M.B. and Huberman, A.M. (1994), *Qualitative Data Analysis*, Second Edition, Sage Publications Ltd., London.

Mutizwa-Mangiza, D. (1988), *An Evaluation of the Effectiveness of Workers' Participation in Decision-making in a Zimbabwean Parastatal Enterprise: A Case Study of the Harare Dairy*, Unpublished MSc Dissertation, University of Zimbabwe, Harare.

Mutizwa-Mangiza, D. (1991), *Staff Retention in the Ministry of Health*, Unpublished report, Government of Zimbabwe, Harare.

Navarro, V. (1988), 'Professional Dominance or Proletarianisation?: Neither', *The Milbank Quarterly*, 66 (Supplement 2), pp. 57-75.

Nyaruwata, O.I. (1988), 'Macro-economic Management, Adjustment and Stabilisation', in C. Stoneman (ed), *Zimbabwe's Prospects*, pp. 90-117, Macmillan, London.

Oppenheimer, M. (1973), 'Proletarianisation of the Professional', *Sociological Review Monograph*, 20, pp. 213-227.

Philips, D.L. (1971), *Knowledge From What?*, Rand McNally and Company, Chicago.

Phimister, I. (1988), 'The Combined and Contradictory Inheritance of the Struggle against Colonialism', in C. Stoneman (ed), *Zimbabwe's Prospects*, pp. 8-15, Macmillan Publishers, London.

Plummer, K. (1983), *Documents of Life*, Unwin Hyman, London.

Punch, M. (1986), *The Politics and Ethics of Field Work*, Sage Publications, London.

Renzetti, C.M. and Lee, R.M. (1993), 'The Problems of Researching Sensitive Topics', in C.M. Renzetti and R.M. Lee (eds), *Researching Sensitive Topics*, Sage Publications, London.

Riddell, R. (1980), *Report on The Commission of Inquiry into Incomes, Prices and Conditions of Service*, Government Printers, Harare.

Riska, E. 'The Professional Status of Physicians in the Nordic Countries' *The Milbank Quarterly*, 66 (Supplement 2), pp. 134-147.

Robinson, J. (1989), *A Patient Voice at the GMC: A Lay Members View of the General Medical Council*, Health Rights.

Roemer, I.R. (1986), 'Proletarianisation of Physicians or Organization of Health Services', *International Journal of Health Services*, 16 (3), pp. 469-477.

Rosenthal, M.M. (1987), *Dealing with Medical Malpractice: The British and Swedish Experience*, Tavistock, London.

Rosenthal, M.M. (1995), *The Incompetent Doctor: Behind Closed Doors*, Open University Press, Buckingham.

Rosenthal, M.M. (1988), 'Medical Discipline in Cross-cultural Perspective: The United States, Britain and Sweden', in R. Dingwall and P. Fenn (eds), *Quality and Regulation in Health Care*, pp. 26-50, Routledge, London.

Rothman, D.J. and Rothman, S.M. (1992), 'A Death in Zimbabwe', *New York Review of Books*, pp. 21-24.

Sachikonye, L.M. (1987), 'State, Capital and Labour', in I. Mandaza (ed), *Zimbabwe: The Political Economy of Transition 1980-1987*, pp. 243-274, CODESRIA, Kent.

Saks, M. (1995), 'The Changing Response of the Medical Profession to Alternative Medicine in Britain: a case of altruism or self-interest?', in T. Johnson, G. Larkin and M. Saks (eds), *Health Professions and the State in Europe*, pp. 103-115, Routledge, London.

Saks, M. (1994), 'The alternatives to medicine', in J. Gabe, D. Kelleher and G. Williams (eds), *Challenging Medicine*, pp. 84-103, Routledge, London.

Sanders, D. (1990), 'Equity in Health: Zimbabwe Nine Years On', *Journal of Social Change in Africa*, 5 (1), pp. 5-22.

Scott, J. (1990), *A Matter of Record*, Polity Press, Cambridge.

Schatzman, L. and Strauss, A.L. (1973), *Field Research: Strategies for a Natural Sociology*, Prentice-Hall, Englewood Cliffs.

Shaw, T. (1988), 'State of Crisis: International Constraints, Contradictions and Capitalism?' in D. Rothchild and N. Chazan (eds), *The Precarious Balance: State and Society in Africa*, pp. 307-324, Westview Press Inc., Boulder.

Sibanda, A. (1988), 'The Political Situation', in C. Stoneman (ed), *Zimbabwe's Prospects*, pp. 257-283, Macmillan Publishers, London.

Silverman, D. (1985), *Qualitative Methodology and Sociology*, Gower, Aldershot.

Sithole, M. (1991), 'Should Zimbabwe Go Where Others Are Coming From?', in I. Mandaza and L.M. Sachikonye (eds), *The One Party State and Democracy*, pp. 71-82, Southern Africa Political Economy (SAPES) Trust, Harare.

Spencer, G. (1982), 'Methodological Issues in the Study of Bureaucratic Elites: A Case Study of West Point', in R.G. Burgess (ed), *Field Research: A Sourcebook and Manual*, pp. 23-25, Routledge, London.

Spradley, J. (1979), *The Ethnographic Interview*, Rinehart & Winston, New York.

Summerton, N. (1995), 'Positive and Negative Factors in Defensive Medicine: A Questionnaire Study of General Practitioners', *British Medical Journal*, 310, pp. 27-29.

Stacey, M. (1969), *Methods of Social Research*, Pergamon, Oxford.

Stacey, M. (1988), *The Sociology of Health and Healing*, Unwin and Unwin, London.

Stacey, M. (1992), *Regulating British Medicine*, John Wiley and Sons, Chichester.

Starr, P. (1982), *The Social Transformation of American Medicine*, Basic Books Inc. Publishers, New York.

Stolfus Jost, T. (1992), 'Recent Developments in Medical Quality Assurance and Audit: an International Comparative Study', in R. Dingwall and P. Fenn (eds), *Quality and Regulation of Health Care*, pp. 69-88, Routledge, London.

Stone, D.A. (1980), *The Limits of Professional Power*, The University of Chicago Press, Chicago.

Stoneman, C. (1988), 'The Economy: Recognising the Reality', in C. Stoneman (ed), *Zimbabwe's Prospects*, pp. 43-62, Macmillan, London.

Strauss, L. A. (1987), *Qualitative Analysis for Social Scientists*, Cambridge University Press, Cambridge.

Tordoff, W. (1984), *Government and Politics in Africa*, Macmillan, London.

Tremblay, M. (1982), 'The Key Informant Technique: A Non-Ethnographic Application', in R.G. Burgess (ed), *Field Research: A Sourcebook and Field Manual*, pp. 98-104, Routledge, London.

Ushewokunze, H.S.M. (1984), *An Agenda for Zimbabwe*, College Press, Harare.

Van Onselen, C. (1976), *Chibaro*, Pluto Press, London.

Watkins, S.(1987), *Medicine and Labour: The Politics of a Profession*, Lawrence and Wishort, London.

Wand, S. and Mekie, E.C. (1957), *Central African Journal of Medicine*, October, pp. 422-423.

Wand, S. and Mekie, E.C. (1958), 'Report of Visit to Central African Branches of B.M.A.', *Central African Journal of Medicine*, April, pp. 178-189.

Weber, M. (1978), *Economy and Society: An Outline of Interpretive Sociology*, University of California Press, Berkeley.

Webster, M.H. (1972), 'A Review of the Development of the Health Services of Rhodesia from 1923 to the Present Day', *Central African Journal of Medicine*, 18 (12), pp. 244-247; 19 (1), pp. 7-9; and 19 (2), pp. 27-51.

Webster, M.H. (1973), 'Whither Medicine in Rhodesia?', *Central African Journal of Journal of Medicine*, 19 (11), pp. 229-234.

Whyte, W.F. (1982), 'Interviewing in Field Research', in R.G. Burgess (ed), *Field Research: A Sourcebook and Field Manual*, pp. 111-122. Routledge, London.

Witz, A. (1994), 'The Challenge of Nursing', in J. Gabe, D. Kelleher and G. Williams (eds), *Challenging Medicine*, pp. 23-45, Routledge, London.

Wolinsky, F.D. (1988), 'The Professional Dominance Perspective Revisited' *The Milbank Quarterly*, 66 (Supplement 2), pp. 33-47.

Wolinsky, F.D. (1993), 'The Professional Dominance, Deprofessionalisation, Proletarianisation, and Corporatisation Perspectives: An Overview and Synthesis', in F.W. Hafferty and J.B. McKinlay (eds), *The Changing Medical Profession*, pp. 11-24, Oxford University Press, Oxford.

Yates, J. (1995), *Private Eye, Heart and Hip*, Churchill Livingstone, Edinburgh.

Young, C. (1988), 'The African Colonial State and its Political Legacy', in D. Rothchild and N. Chazan (eds), *The Precarious Balance: State and Society in Africa*, pp. 25-67, Westview Press Inc., Boulder.

Zola, I.K. (1972), 'Medicine as an Institution of Social Control', *The Sociological Review*, 20, pp. 487-503.

Government and Parliamentary Publications and Reports

Government of Southern Rhodesia, (1925), *Public Health Act (Chapter 386)*, Government Printers, Salisbury.

Government of Southern Rhodesia, (1927), Notice 335, 17 June.

Government of Southern Rhodesia, (1938), *Secretary's Report on the Public Health for the Year 1937*, Government Printers, Harare.

Government of Southern Rhodesia, (1946), *Commission of Enquiry into the National Health Services Report*, also known as the Saints Commission, Government Printers, Salisbury.

Government of Southern Rhodesia, Undated, *Rules and Regulations for the Management of Government Hospitals*, Government Printers, Salisbury.

Federal Government of Rhodesia and Nyasaland, (1960), *Report of the Commission of Enquiry into the Health and Medical Services of the Federation*, also known as the Morton Commission, Government Printers, Salisbury.

Government of Rhodesia, (1963), *Secretary's Report on the Public Health for the Year 1962*, Government Printers, Salisbury.

Government of Zimbabwe, (1971), *Medical Dental and Allied Professions Act (Chapter 224)*, Government Printers, Harare.

Government of Rhodesia, (1975), *Salisbury Hospitals Act (No. 16)*, Government Printers, Salisbury.

Government of Rhodesia-Zimbabwe, (1979), *The Medical Services Act* (No. 7), Government Printers, Salisbury.

Government of Zimbabwe, (1981), *National Manpower Survey*, Government Printers, Harare.

Government of Zimbabwe, Ministry of Health, (1984), *Planning for Equity in Health: A Sectoral Review Statement*, Government Printers, Harare.

Government of Zimbabwe, Ministry of Health, (1987), *Drugs and Allied Substances Control Amendment Act*, Government Printers, Harare.

Government of Zimbabwe, (1989), *Report of the Public Service Review Commission of Zimbabwe*, under the chairmanship of Professor D. Kavran, Government Printers, Harare.

Government of Zimbabwe, *Public Service (Maintenance of Services), Regulations, 1990*, (Statutory Instrument 258, 1990).

Government of Zimbabwe, (1990), *A Decade of Implementing Health For All Strategies: A Zimbabwean Experience (1980-1989)*, Unpublished report.

Government of Zimbabwe, (1992), *Public Service (Disciplinary) Regulations (Statutory Instrument 125 of 1992)*, Government Printers, Harare.

Government of Zimbabwe, (1992), *Public Services (Disciplinary) Regulations (Statutory Instrument 65 of 1992*, Government Printers, Harare.

Government of Zimbabwe, (1992), *Public/Private Sector for Health Care Study Consultative Meeting: Proceedings of the First Consultative Meeting, 6-7 October*, Unpublished report.

Government of Zimbabwe, (1993), *Medical Dental and Allied Professions (Information) Regulations (Chapter 224)*, (Statutory Instrument 93 of 1993).

Government of Zimbabwe, Ministry of Health and Child Welfare, (1994), *Policy and Management Options for Parirenyatwa Group of Hospitals: Report of the Technical Committee*, Unpublished report.

Government of Zimbabwe, (1995), *Health Sector Reform in Zimbabwe*, Concept Paper on Decentralisation in the Ministry of Health and Child Welfare.

Parliament of Zimbabwe, *Parliamentary Debates*, 26 March, 1987.

Parliament of Zimbabwe, *Parliamentary Debates*, 31 March, 1987.

Parliament of Zimbabwe, *Parliamentary Debates*, 21 November, 1990.

Parliament of Zimbabwe, *First Report of the Service Ministries Committee on the Ministry of Health*, Vote No. 15-1990-91.

Parliament of Zimbabwe, Vote No. 14-1992-93.

Parliament of Zimbabwe, *Parliamentary Debates*, 19 March, 1992.

Parliament of Zimbabwe, *Parliamentary Debates*, 20 October, 1993.

Parliament of Zimbabwe, *Second Interim Report of the Parliamentary Select Committee on the Functioning of the Health Professions Council*, 20 October, 1993.

Parliament of Zimbabwe, *Parliamentary Debates*, 2 March, 1993.

Parliament of Zimbabwe, *Parliamentary Debates*, 2 November, 1993.

Parliament of Zimbabwe, *Parliamentary Debates*, 3 November, 1993.

Parliament of Zimbabwe, *Parliamentary Debates*, 6 November, 1993.

Parliament of Zimbabwe (1995), *Report of the Comptroller and Auditor General on the Ministry of Health and Child Welfare on Casualty, Out-patients, Maternity Departments (Central and Provincial Hospitals), and Manpower Utilisation.*

Unpublished Reports, Memoranda and Letters

College of Primary Care Physicians and Pharmaceutical Society, 'Ethics Conference', Kadoma, November, 1992.
Document presented to the Minister of Health and Child Welfare by the Hospital Doctors Association on 18 February, 1994.
Letter from the Hospital Doctors' Association to the Minister of Health dated 8 March, 1994.
Letter from Provincial Medical Director of Health Care Services, Ministry of Health and Child Welfare, to the Hospital Doctors Association, dated 29 March, 1994.
University of Zimbabwe, *New Medical Curriculum Review*, 1992.
Health Professions Council, 1993, *Health Professions Council Functions and a Guide to Ethics*, unpublished.
Zimbabwe Nurses Association President's letter to Hospital Doctors Association's President dated 25 April, 1994.
Zimbabwe Nurses Association President's letter to state President dated 26 April, 1994.
Zimbabwe Medical Association Newsletter, 1992.
Zimbabwe Medical Association Constitution, undated.
Health Professions Council, *Health Professions Council Functions and A Guide to Ethics*, Harare, 1993 (Unpublished document).

National Newspapers and Magazines

'Doctors Can't Hold Nation to Ransom', in *Chronicle*, 11 December, 1988.
'McGowan Wins Court Case', in *Daily Gazette*, 13 January, 1994.
Financial Gazette, 11 May, 1995.
Financial Gazette, 16 June, 1994.
Herald, 20 December, 1980.
'Minister Attacks Parasite Doctors', in *Herald*, 8 October, 1981.
'Warning to State Doctors', in *Herald*, 18 September, 1982.
Herald, 24 July, 1984.

Herald, 10 January, 1984.

Herald, 8 December, 1984.

Herald, 18 April, 1985.

'Improve Pay for Doctors', in *Herald*, 6 March 1987.

'Doctors Urged to Abandon Strike', in *Herald*, 13 November, 1988.

'Threat to Strike: Doctors Warned of Heavy Penalty', in *Herald*, 6 December, 1988.

'Why Junior Doctors Feel Like Going on Strike', in *Herald*, 11 December, 1988.

'Doctors Return to Work after 3 Day Strike', in *Herald*, 15 December, 1988.

'ZCTU Backs Doctors Strike, But ...', in *Herald*, 15 December, 1988.

'Harare Team Geared for Open Heart Ops as Machines Arrive', in *Sunday Mail*, 12 February, 1989.

'Doctors Say No to Sweeping Powers for Minister', in *Herald*, 18 May, 1989.

'Ministry Replies to ZIMA', in *Herald*, 19 May, 1989.

'Junior Doctors Oppose Bill', in *Herald*, 25 May, 1989.

Herald, 13 June, 1989.

Herald, 16 June, 1989.

Herald, 15 June, 1989.

'Stamps Appeals for End to Laxity at Hospital', in *Herald*, 25 September, 1990.

'Critics of Doctors Stamped on by Stamps', in *The Herald*, 23 November, 1990.

'Out-dated Medical Equipment Common', in *Herald*, 8 November, 1990.

'ZMA Announces System to Monitor Doctors Conduct', in *Herald*, 4 March, 1993.

'Nation Faces Shortage of Speech Therapists', in *Herald*, 11 March, 1993.

'McGowan Allowed to Practise', in *Herald*, 17 July, 1993.

'Critical Shortage of Physiotherapists', in *Herald*, 5 September, 1993.

'UZ Students Fast over McGowan', in *Herald*, 19 October, 1993.

Herald, 20 October, 1993.

'Breakthrough Reached with Striking Doctors', in *Herald*, 20 April, 1994

'No Settlement Yet in Strike by Junior Doctors', in *Herald*, 21 April, 1994.

'Return to Work or You are Fired', in *Herald*, 25, April, 1994.

Herald, 29 May, 1994.

Herald, 10 June, 1994.

'Doctors Should not Blackmail State', in *Herald*, 5 May, 1994.

'State's Position on Sacked Doctors', in *Herald*, 4 May, 1994.

Herald, 12 May, 1995.

'Health Ministry Fails to Discipline Doctors', in *Herald*, 18 May, 1995.

Herald, 22 May, 1995

'Ministry's Financial Crisis Reaches New Proportions', in *Herald*, 3 February, 1996.

'Shot in the Arm for Ministry', in *Herald*, 25 January, 1996.

Horizon, March/April, 1995.

Horizon, June, 1995.

Northern News, October, 1993.

'Hospitals a National Disaster', in *Sunday Mail*, 2 January, 1994.

'Better Incentives Needed for Medical Personnel', in *Sunday Gazette*, 16 May, 1993.

Sunday Mail, 5 March, 1995.

Sunday Mail, 31 March, 1985.

Sunday Mail, 29 May, 1994.

Students Union, 18 October, 1993.

Sunday Mail, 29 May, 1994.

Sunday Mail, 15 May, 1994.

'Indiscipline May Wreck Hospitals', in *Herald*, 16 August, 1983.

'The McGowan Case: Was Parliamentary Committee Ignored', in *ZimRights News*, December, 1993.

'McGowan Trial - Relevant Witnesses Not Called by AG', in *ZimRights News*, May/June, 1994.

ZimRights News, October, 1995.

'Irregularities in the Preparation for the trial of Dr Richard Gladwell McGowan', in *ZimRights News*, 17 May, 1994.

Appendix

Members of the Health Professions Council

1. The Secretary for Health
2. The following ten members appointed by the Minister of Health:
    a. A Medical Practitioner who is a member of the Faculty of Medicine, University of Zimbabwe
    b. Registered legal practitioner with at least five years experience
    c. A registered medical practitioner
    d. A registered dental practitioner
    e. A registered pharmaceutical chemist
    f. A registered general nurse
    g. One other person from any other professional group not mentioned above
    h. Two persons who are not registered but selected by the Minister of Health for their suitability to the Council
    i. A representative of the Missions in Zimbabwe selected by the Minister of Health
3. Sixteen persons elected by members of their profession
    a. Two registered medical practitioners elected by registered medical practitioners
    b. A registered dental practitioner
    c. A registered pharmaceutical chemist
    d. Seven nurses of which not less than 2 should be state certified nurses
    e. A registered environmental health officer or technician
    f. Two registered medical laboratory technologists or registered state certified medical laboratory technologists or state certified medical laboratory technicians
    g. One psychologist
    h. One health professional from any registered profession not covered above

Index of Authors Cited

General Index

abortion 135
accountability 141, 163, 208, 234
achievements of post-independence government in health care provision 105, 109
Africa Health 127
Africa Watch 212
Africanisation 28
aid programmes 105, 218, 231, 233, 236–7
AIDS 126, 132, 185
alternative therapies 17; *see also* traditional medicine
American Medical Association (AMA) 5, 18, 206
ancestral spirits 139
Andrew Fleming Hospital *see* Parirenyatwa Hospital
anonymity of research respondents 52, 66–7
antibiotics 120–21
Dr Askins 90
Attorney General's Office 204–5, 211, 224
audit system *see* medical audit
autonomy, medical
 definition of 6–8
 dimensions and degrees of 11, 20
 erosion of 9–15, 97, 112–14, 118, 121, 130–31, 134, 136–8, 153, 161, 163, 169, 174–5, 225–31 *passim*, 237

in diagnosing 114–18
in prescribing 119–22, 219
in regulation of medical education, registration and discipline 180, 191, 222–3
in treatment 122–7
of doctors at different levels 176–7
political 96
proposed model of 217, 227, 233–7
see also clinical autonomy; collective autonomy; economic autonomy
autopsy reports 204, 210–11
Avenues Clinic 210, 212, 214

barium meals 117
Bill of Rights 25
biographies as data sources 61–2
Dr Blair 85
'bonding' contract 5, 97, 103, 145, 147–50, 157, 221
boycotting of classes by students 155
breast cancer 12–13
Britain 3–9, 13–20, 24–5, 104, 113–14, 125, 130–31, 135–44 *passim*, 175, 179, 191–3, 213, 220, 224–9 *passim*, 234, 237
British Medical Association (BMA) 5, 74, 84, 86–9, 91–3, 96, 198–9, 218, 226
British South Africa Company 70–71, 82, 84

cardiac treatment 127
career structure for government

self-regulation 18–19, 198
formal and informal 179–80
shared posts for doctors 100, 122
sharing of beds 110
shortages *see* doctors; drugs; equipment; nurses
social development programme 29–31
Social Dimension of Adjustment Fund (SDF) and SDF patients 107–9, 115–16, 120, 131, 162–3, 219–20
socialist political agenda 28–31
South Africa 27, 90, 127, 147–8, 168, 189
Stamps, Timothy 50, 157, 169, 211
state, the
definition of 20
role of 6, 9–10
status of doctors 143, 146–7, 161, 182, 227–8
Statutory Instrument 93 (1993) 134–6, 139, 141, 196–7, 200, 209, 212, 215
Statutory Instrument 258 (1990) 166
sterilization of equipment 56
strike by laboratory technicians 173
strikes by doctors
in 1984 163–73 *passim*
in 1988 1, 144, 150
in 1989 150, 154–7, 168, 170–71, 177
in 1994 50–52, 55, 64–8 *passim*, 163, 165–71, 173, 188, 198, 208

prohibited by contract 111, 167, 171
structural adjustment programmes *see* economic structural adjustment programmes
student demonstrations 155, 211, 213
subsidies for health care 72, 74, 106
surgeons-in-charge 81
Sweden 20, 135–6, 181, 193, 197, 201–3, 207

tape-recording of interviews 52–3
tax exemptions 74, 89, 95, 101, 158, 218
teaching hospitals 122–3
testing, diagnostic, facilities for 117–18, 132, 140, 173, 219
thyroid function tests 117
timetabling of doctors' work 160
traditional medicine 4, 75, 77–9, 89, 95, 97, 229
legalisation of 100, 174–5, 202
training of doctors *see* medical education
triangulation 37, 57, 63–4
turnover of doctors 1, 144–6, 157–8, 176, 221
turnover of Ministers and Secretaries for Health 177

Ultra sound equipment 117
Umtali Mission 77
undercharging for health services 72, 74, 106, 218, 221, 235
unilateral declaration of independence 22
United Bulawayo Central Hospitals 94

United States 5–9, 13–20, 24–5, 40, 81, 113–14, 130, 135–41, 179, 199–200, 220–30 *passim*, 234, 237
University of Birmingham 102, 188
University of Zimbabwe 102, 185–8, 198

victims' organisations 208

'Willowgate Scandal' 33
'witch hunting' through medical audit 129
Witchcraft Suppression Act (1899) 4, 77, 89
women, attitudes to and treatment of 12–13, 59, 66
women doctors 111
World Bank 105–7, 121–2, 219, 235–6
World Health Organisation 103

X-ray services 56, 109, 115, 118

Zambia 3, 22, 24–6, 62, 80
Zimbabwe, map of 23
Zimbabwe African National Union (ZANU) 24–7, 98
Zimbabwe African People's Union (ZAPU) 24–5
Zimbabwe Congress of Trade Unions (ZCTU) 109, 150, 155, 173
Zimbabwe Medical Association 60, 93, 96, 111–12, 119, 128–9, 135–6, 150–53, 158, 164, 170, 198, 206–7, 209, 226
Zimbabwe National Traditional Healers' Association (ZINATHA) 100
Zimbabwe Nurses' Association 60, 152, 182–4
reactions to doctors' strike 171–2
Zimbabwe Teachers Association 173
ZimRights News 209